PHARMACOLOGY

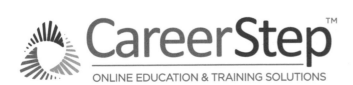

ONLINE EDUCATION & TRAINING SOLUTIONS

Career Step, LLC
Phone: 801.489.9393
Toll-Free: 800.246.7837
Fax: 801.491.6645
careerstep.com

This text companion contains a snapshot of the online program content converted to a printed format. Please note that the online training program is constantly changing and improving and is always the source of the most up-to-date information.

Product Number: HG-PR-11-006
Generation Date: March 13, 2015

TABLE OF CONTENTS

UNIT 1
Introduction

INTRODUCTION TO PHARMACOLOGY

Learning Objectives

Pharmacology Basics – Students will be able to distinguish between different categories of drugs and their basic actions and effects.

Drug Administration – Students will be able to distinguish between different topical, enteral, and parenteral administration routes.

Drug Categories and Functions – Students will be able to properly identify common drugs and their basic functions from the following categories: cardiovascular, digestive, endocrine, immune, pain management, psychological, and respiratory.

Drug References – Students will be able to use legitimate resources to find drug definitions, dosages, pronunciations, and other related information.

Prescription Interpretation – Students will be able to properly interpret medications, dosages, and instructions for medication administration.

Medication Spelling Accuracy – Students will be able to correctly spell commonly prescribed medications.

If you go to most any dictionary, you find a number of words that begin with the prefix *pharma-*, from the Greek *pharmakon*, which means drug. **Pharmacology**, then, is more or less the study of drugs. So, what is a drug? In a general sense, it is any substance (with the notable exception of food) intended to affect the structure or function of any part of the human body (or other animals). Think about that. It's a broad definition that incorporates the different ways that we think of "drugs" in our society. Let's talk specifically about a few of those:

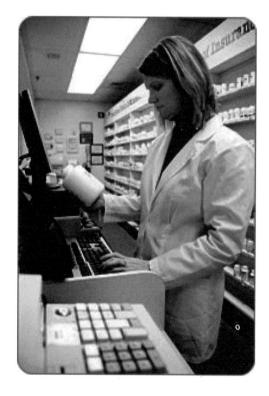

1. Any chemical compound used on or administered to humans or animals as an aid in the diagnosis, treatment, or prevention of disease or other abnormal condition, for the relief of pain or suffering, or to control or improve any physiologic or pathologic condition.
2. A chemical substance that affects the processes of the mind or body.
3. A substance used recreationally for its effects on the central nervous system, such as a narcotic; its abuse may lead to dependence or addiction.

A **drug** can be something that occurs naturally in our environment or can be synthetically created in a laboratory. Drugs in some form or another have been a component of every society throughout recorded history. In Western medicine particularly, drugs are a primary method of treating illness and disease. Of course you know this. Most people only go to the doctor when they absolutely have to in order to get a drug (or medical procedure) that could not otherwise be obtained, such as an antibiotic. Given their prevalence as a method of treatment, it should be no surprise to you that they will appear in virtually every medical record that you edit. They are prescribed in clinic notes, used during surgeries, listed and discussed as part of H&Ps, consultations, discharge summaries, and emergency room records. They are used in diagnostic reports as a means of performing procedures.

With all of these applications, there are quite literally thousands of different types of drugs. There is good news, though. As a medical transcription editor you will never have to prescribe or administer drugs to patients! What that means is that you will not need to learn everything there is to know about pharmacology. You won't need to be able to diagnose, determine the appropriate medication for a number of pathologies, anesthetize a patient, or be concerned with how various drugs may interact with each other.

What will you need to know as a medical transcription editor?

Drugs are classified in some general ways and have consistencies in their naming, which are common to virtually all drugs. It is also useful to know the different ways that drugs get assimilated into the body, especially as those terms relate to medical reports.

In practical application, drugs get grouped into a variety of different types based on what it is that they do within the body. Do they lower fever? Stop the blood from clotting? Help you sleep? These general groupings appear over and over again in medical reports. There are several individual drugs that would appropriately be represented in these groups. The more drugs with which you are familiar, the easier it will be for you to recognize, locate, and accurately spell them when you begin transcription editing. Gaining an understanding of what types of drugs exist and what they are used for will help when you invariably come across garbled dictation and have to determine a particular medication through context. Learning how to use good reference tools (books and online) will help with this as well.

Finally, if you have ever looked at a prescription given to you by your doctor, you are well aware that it is not written in plain English. There are a variety of (mostly foreign) terms employed by physicians to represent dosages and instructions. As an MTE, you will need to know what these are and how to edit them accurately.

UNIT 2
Pharmacology Basics

PHARMACOLOGY BASICS – INTRODUCTION

In this pharmacology basics unit we will cover the fundamentals of pharmaceuticals—must-know information for anyone working in the medical industry.

Specifically, this unit will cover:

- **Types of Drugs**
- **Drug Effect**
- **Drug Treatment**

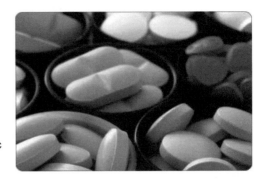

You will not be required to memorize all the information in this pharmacology module, but having a firm understanding of how drugs work, how they are named, and their basic functions will help you tremendously as you edit medical records.

TWO TYPES OF DRUGS

As far as the classifications of drugs go, first and foremost, in the United States drugs are categorized by law into two main groups:

- prescription drugs
- over-the-counter drugs (also called OTC drugs)

Prescription drugs require the written authorization of a licensed medical professional, a physician, dentist, physician's assistant, or nurse practitioner, to name a few. The Federal Government has enacted a law that states these types of drugs are considered safe for people to use only under direct medical supervision. In order to procure these drugs, it is necessary to get an "order" from a practitioner, called a **prescription**.

Prescription drugs have a subcategory known as **controlled substances**. Because some drugs that are useful in the practice of medicine also have a potential for abuse, dependence, or addiction, there are government controls in place to even more carefully regulate their production, distribution, and use. These prescription drugs, known as controlled substances, are usually things like narcotics, stimulants, and tranquilizers.

In fact, the regulation and oversight of drugs in the United States involves a number of federal agencies and an enormous amount of money. Before a new drug ever finds its way into your doctor's hands (or your body), it undergoes an extensive research and testing process, lengthy approval procedures, and ongoing reporting, consumer advocacy, and legal control processes. The Drug Enforcement Administration (DEA), the Department of Health and Human Services, the Food and Drug Administration, and the Attorney General are all involved. Local and federal police departments and the Department of Justice provide enforcement of the controls put in place by the government.

On the other hand, nonprescription or over-the-counter drugs do not require written authorization and can be purchased without restriction—well, pretty much without restriction. In recent years, the purchase of *pseudoephedrine*, an ingredient in common cold medicines, has started to be limited because of its use in the illegal production of methamphetamine. It's now classified as a "behind-the-counter" drug that can only be purchased in limited quantities. On the other hand, historically, if a regulated drug proves to be safe after years of widespread use, restrictions can be lifted and such a drug can be sold over the counter. An example of one such drug is *ibuprofen*, a drug that reduces pain, fever, and inflammation. For years ibuprofen was available only with a prescription, but it is now an OTC drug with a maximum allowable potency of 200 mg. Ibuprofen in large dosages (up to 800 mg) is still regulated.

Highlights

Prescription drugs include controlled substances. Controlled substances are categorized in a 1–5 schedule system, with schedule 1 having the highest potential for addiction/abuse and schedule 5 having the lowest potential for addiction/abuse. Examples of schedule I drugs include:

- marijuana
- LSD
- heroin

Because they are not considered safe, these cannot be prescribed.

The FDA has recently (October 2007) proposed adding a third class of drug: behind-the-counter (BTC). These would be available without a prescription but only by requesting them directly from a pharmacist. There are many countries that currently offer BTC drugs, including Australia, Canada, Germany, and the United Kingdom.

Multiple Choice.
Choose the best answer.

1. _____ drugs are available for unregulated purchase at many stores.

   ○ Prescription

   ○ Over-the-counter

   ○ Behind-the-counter

2. Ibuprofen, 200 mg, is an example of a/an _____ medication.

   ○ prescription

   ○ over-the-counter

   ○ behind-the-counter

3. A new class of drug is _____ drugs, which means that these drugs can be purchased without a prescription but must be requested from the pharmacist.

   ○ prescription

   ○ over-the-counter

   ○ behind-the-counter

4. Antibiotics are _____ drugs, so they are only available from a pharmacist with direction from a physician.

   ○ prescription

   ○ over-the-counter

   ○ behind-the-counter

5. New laws only allow the purchase of limited quantities of pseudoephedrine, and it is classified as a _____ drug.

   ○ prescription

   ○ over-the-counter

   ○ behind-the-counter

DRUG NAMES

How drugs are named presents a peculiar problem to medical transcription editors. Drug names are among the more challenging aspects of the language of medicine. There are a couple of reasons for this, and one reason is that a drug has more than one name associated with it.

In fact, most drugs have three names (at least):

1. A chemical name.
2. A generic name, also called a nonproprietary name.
3. A brand name, also called a proprietary or trade name.

The **chemical** name is precisely that: the atomic or molecular structure of the drug. The chemical name can be simple—as in sodium bicarbonate, potassium chloride, or calcium. Likewise, it can be very complex—as in 7-chloro-1,3-dihydro-1-methyl-5-phenyl-2H-1,4-benzodiazepin-2-one, which is the chemical name for **Valium**, a drug used to treat anxiety. Luckily for us, the chemical name is rarely used in medical reports because it is so often long and cumbersome.

Drugs are generally developed by publicly-held companies. Those companies will spend years creating and testing a drug, and then several more years getting it FDA approved, making it legal to market and distribute the drug for a specific purpose. When a drug company receives approval for its product, it also receives a patent on the unique chemical composition that comprises that drug. Eventually, those patents expire. When they do, the proprietary name the drug company gave to that drug continues to be owned by that drug company. However, a **generic name** is adopted for the drug. At that point, other companies can manufacture it, using the same chemical composition. The generic name assigned to the drug is an official name approved in the U.S. by an organization called the United States Adopted Names (USAN) Council.

Drugs can have at least three names:

- Chemical
- Generic
- Brand or Trade

All generic names must be unique. By FDA rules, any generic versions of a given drug—no matter what company manufactures it—must have the same active ingredients and be absorbed into the body at the same rate. A generic drug name may or may not reflect the chemical name, structure, or formula. Refer to the same example used above. The generic name for Valium is **diazepam**, which does partially reflect the chemical structure (1,4-benzodiazepin). By the same token, the generic name for Glucophage is **metformin**, a drug used in the treatment of diabetes. Its chemical name is N,N-dimethylimidodicarbonimidic diamide hydrochloride. The generic name is not in any way related to the chemical name. For transcription editing purposes, it doesn't really matter one way or the other whether it is related to the chemical name or not.

The third name given to a drug is the **brand** (or trade) **name**, and it is the name selected by a manufacturer for its particular product. The same generic drug (with the same chemical composition) may be produced by several pharmaceutical companies and marketed under different names. For example, ibuprofen is sold as Advil, Motrin, Genpril, Nuprin, Menadol, and Ibu-Tab, among others. Brand or trade names are the names you read in magazine ads and see on TV commercials: Nexium, Viagra, Allegra, Tylenol, Motrin, Celebrex, Fosamax, Zantac, Naprosyn, and, of course, hundreds of others.

The important thing to know about brand names is that in medical reports they are always capitalized. Generic drugs, however, are only capitalized if they begin a sentence or if they are part of a numbered list.

The following chart shows some commonly used drugs with their chemical, generic, and brand names.

Chemical Name	Generic Name	Brand Name
N-(4-hydroxyphenyl) acetamide	acetaminophen	Tylenol
cephalosporin C (antibiotic)	cephalexin	Keflex
acetylsalicylic acid	aspirin*	Bufferin
potassium chloride	potassium chloride	Kay Ciel
N-methyl-3-phenyl-3-[4-(trifluoromethyl)phenoxy]propan-1-amine	fluoxetine hydrochloride	Prozac

*Aspirin is an example of a brand name for a preparation originally developed by the Bayer company that has come to be a generic name and used to refer to any product having the same chemistry.

Terminology.

Enter each term in the space provided. Read the definition and description for each term.

1. chemical name _____

The name given for the atomic or molecular structure of a drug.

2. Valium _____

Tranquilizer. Used to treat anxiety.

3. generic name _____

The name given a drug which is NOT a proprietary name, but the name which is used by any manufacturer.

4. diazepam _____

The generic name for Valium, an antianxiety medication.

5. metformin _____

The generic name for a medication which lowers blood sugar levels. Used in the treatment of diabetes.

6. brand name _____

A manufacturer's proprietary name for their medication. It is always capitalized.

Multiple Choice.

Choose the best answer.

1. Drugs can have at least (○ three, ○ five) different types of names.

2. The first letter of a brand name drug is (○ never, ○ always) capitalized.

3. The chemical name of a drug is (○ rarely, ○ often) used in medical reports.

4. Drugs can have multiple (○ trade or brand, ○ generic) names.

5. The first letter of a generic drug is (○ always, ○ never) capitalized within a sentence.

NAMING CHALLENGE

Let's go back to the explanation about how a drug comes to be. The company that develops and gets the first patent on a drug also earns the right to name it. Once the patent expires on that drug and any company can manufacture it, each company also has the right to name its marketed version. This makes drugs troublesome to learn.

With the exception of its chemical name—which we have already established is not used—there is simply no rhyme or reason to how a drug is named. You may remember that the medical language tends to be based on Greek and Latin. As such, it follows a series of rules that make it fairly easy to identify terms and patterns and even commit to memory the meanings of individual word parts. This is absolutely not true when it comes to drugs. In fact, to make their version of a drug stand out, companies often use a "cutesy" name or spelling so that their drug name is more memorable. For example, Sine-Aid is a brand name nasal decongestant—aids your sinuses, get it?

While the Internet is a fantastic place to locate and verify drugs, it is a good idea to cross-reference the spelling of a drug using your program resources.

In addition to a lack of consistency in naming and spelling, many drug names sound alike when spoken or look alike on the handwritten or printed page. This can be confusing to the listener or the reader. Medical professionals, when dealing with the selection and documentation of drug therapies, must be especially careful. Your confusion when confronted with these similarities could result in the wrong medication being documented as a permanent part of a patient's chart. Obviously, this is a bad thing.

It is important that you know enough, or know where to go, to determine whether the drug name that you see or hear is, in fact, the correct drug for the context. Potential confusion exists in both generic and brand names, as the following examples clearly demonstrate:

- Banthine (ulcer treatment); Brethine (asthma treatment)
- Capitrol (an antifungal shampoo); captopril (lowers blood pressure)
- desipramine (an antidepressant); deserpidine (lowers blood pressure)
- Procan (heart medicine); procaine (an anesthetic)
- Xanax (anxiety reducer); Zantac (ulcer treatment)

Multiply these examples by a few hundred and you can begin to see the nature of the problem. All professionals in the healthcare process—from those providing direct patient care to those documenting the healthcare process—have the responsibility to be vigilant when choosing, prescribing, spelling, and documenting drugs.

DRUG EFFECT

In order for a drug to do absolutely anything to treat an illness, it has to somehow get into or onto the patient's body. This can be accomplished in a variety of ways, depending on what the desired effect is.

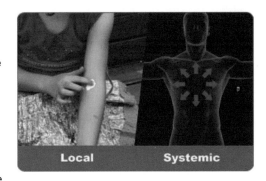

Drugs are given for either a **local** effect or a **systemic** effect. If the desired *effect* of the medication is limited to a specific area of the body, it is defined as local. This doesn't refer to how it is administered but rather to what the goal is of this particular drug. The Novocain your dentist uses to anesthetize a very specific area in your mouth is an example of a drug used to achieve a local effect. Lotion rubbed on dry skin and eye drops applied to itchy, red eyes are also examples of local effect.

On the other hand, if the medication is carried through the blood or skin and then throughout the entire body it is systemic. Again, think of the goal or desired effect of the medication, not the way that it is administered. Imagine that you have a headache. If you take an aspirin orally, the drug will first go to your stomach, where it is absorbed into the bloodstream. It will go to work, making your head feel better. However, because it has a systemic effect, it will take care of that throbbing toe you stubbed as well. Also, if you happen to have a sensitive stomach, it could eliminate the headache and the stubbed toe but give you a tummy ache. In the end, your entire body has experienced the effects of the drug. Taking a medication orally will virtually always result in a systemic effect, because it is absorbed through the stomach and into the bloodstream.

Terminology.
Enter each term in the space provided. Read the definition and description for each term.

1. Local _____

An effect achieved when a drug is administered to a specific area to treat only that area.

2. Systemic _____

An effect achieved when a drug is intended to be assimilated throughout the entire body.

Multiple Choice.
Choose the best answer. Determine whether the following would be examples of a medication having a local effect or systemic effect.

1. Anesthetic applied to the site of a laceration, prior to stitches being applied.

   - local
   - systemic

2. Blood pressure lowering medication, taken orally.

   - local
   - systemic

3. Antifungal cream applied to toenail fungus.

   - local
   - systemic

4. Antibacterial shampoo.

   - local
   - systemic

5. Laxative for constipation.

   - local
   - systemic

DRUG TREATMENT

Medications are given for one of three main purposes: to relieve, cure, or control.

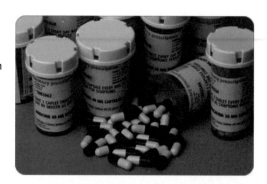

- Taking aspirin for a headache is an example of a drug used to relieve a given condition.
- Taking an antibiotic to clear up a bacterial infection is an example of a medication used to cure.
- Taking insulin to keep blood sugars within proper ranges is an example of a medication used to control.

Following are some examples, taken from actual medical records, of how drugs can be used in the treatment of a patient:

> The patient returns today for a repeat 16 mg Synvisc injection of his left knee. He tolerated the last injection very well and had some significant immediate relief of his pain. He was very happy with his progress after that injection. His left knee was prepped and injected with sterile technique. There were no complications. This was done through the typical inferomedial porthole.

Treatment: Synvisc was used to relieve knee pain.

> The orthopedist ordered the patient to have an injection of 30 mg of Toradol IM for chronic tension headache and injection of 25 mg of Phenergan IM for nausea.

Treatment: Toradol was used to relieve tension headache. Phenergan was used to control nausea.

> The patient's throat culture was positive for strep. We gave her an injection of penicillin, specifically Bicillin L-A 1.2 million units IM.

Treatment: Penicillin was used to cure strep infection.

DRUG ACTION

Regardless of the method of administration, the same general series of processes occurs once the drug enters the body: absorption, distribution, metabolism, and elimination.

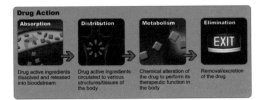

The first of these, **absorption**, is the process by which the active ingredients of a drug preparation are dissolved and released into the bloodstream. Absorption rates vary greatly in terms of time and extent. In the bloodstream, the active ingredients of the drug are circulated to the various structures and tissues of the body. This process is called **distribution**. Once in the body, the drug is either metabolized or excreted, or a combination of the two. In most cases the body chemically alters the drug so it can perform its therapeutic function, and then it is eliminated. The process of chemical alteration is called **metabolism**, and the process of excretion is called **elimination**. Most drugs are metabolized by the liver and excreted through the kidneys. Some excretion, however, occurs through the gastrointestinal tract, or in sweat, saliva, breast milk, and occasionally even exhaled air.

UNIT 3
Administration

ADMINISTRATION – INTRODUCTION

You can determine now whether the effect of a drug is local or systemic. Before a drug can perform its desired effect, however, it has to get into the patient—it has to be administered. **Administration** refers to the various ways drugs are taken or applied. The Food and Drug Administration lists over 100 specific drug administration routes. Some of these methods are familiar to us: swallowing a pill, wearing a patch, or receiving a shot; others are not. We will introduce several drug administration routes in this section.

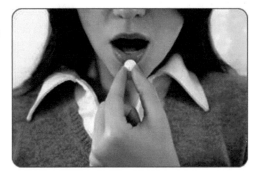

TOPICAL, ENTERAL, AND PARENTERAL

Most methods of administration fit into three broad categories:

Topical: Generally applied directly where action is desired, resulting in a local effect. A transdermal route involves topical application, but is absorbed through the skin resulting in a systemic effect.

Enteral: Applied via the digestive tract; resulting effect is systemic.

Parenteral: Application by any means other than digestive tract, but generally understood as the injectable methods of application. The resulting effect is systemic.

We tend to think of topical as meaning applied to the skin—and usually it is. In general, topical administration has a local effect; however, some medications are absorbed through the skin and have a systemic effect. This is called a **transdermal** route, and includes nicotine patches, nitroglycerin ointment and testosterone ointment, for example.

The term **enteral** quite literally means "relating to or inside the intestines." Although the enteral route is most commonly administered orally, the important factors are that the drugs have a resulting systemic effect and they are absorbed through the digestive tract.

There are many circumstances under which drugs cannot or should not be administered through the digestive tract. In these instances, **parenteral** administration is utilized. The parenteral route has a systemic effect and does not use the gastrointestinal system. It includes most needle injections, including those directly into the veins or arteries, into the muscles, or into the spine. These will be discussed in more detail throughout the remainder of this unit.

Terminology.
Enter each term in the space provided. Read the definition and description for each term.

1. Topical _____

Drug is applied directly to the area where a reaction is desired. The resulting effect is often local.

2. Enteral _____

Drug is applied to the gastrointestinal system. The desired effect is systemic.

3. Parenteral _____

Drug is applied to an area of the body other than the digestive tract. The desired effect is systemic.

Matching.
Match the appropriate terms below.

1. ____ Has a local desired effect.

2. ____ Means "intestinal."

3. ____ Drugs that are generally administered orally.

4. ____ Drugs that are generally administered via injection.

5. ____ Has a systemic effect and is often swallowed.

6. ____ Has a systemic effect and is not swallowed.

7. ____ A nitroglycerin patch uses this type of drug administration.

8. ____ With this type of drug administration, the drug is absorbed into the bloodstream through the stomach and intestines.

A. topical

B. enteral

C. parenteral

D. transdermal

TOPICAL – EARS AND EYES

Some topical administration routes were suggested on the previous page. Let's learn a few of the more common ones, as well as some examples of common medications that are administered via these routes.

Otic

Otic means ear; also called auricular.

Drugs can be administered directly into the ear via a dropper. In fact, the word **drops** is often used in the name of otic medications. Otic drops can be used to treat quite a few medical conditions.

- Carbamide peroxide drops are applied directly into the ear canal to help soften, loosen, and remove earwax.
- Ear infections are often treated via ear drops which may contain a combination of acetic acid, a corticosteroid that relieves redness, itching, and swelling, and an antibiotic to fight the infection.
- A few antibiotics commonly used in otic drops are ciprofloxacin, gentamicin, and neomycin.
- Corticosteroids commonly used in otic drops are dexamethasone, fluocinolone, and hydrocortisone.

Ophthalmic and Ocular

This administration route uses the eyes. Ophthalmic administration usually refers to eye drops. You have probably used these yourself at some point. Intravitreal administration is much less common and is accomplished via a needle into the vitreous of the eye.

Eye drops can be used to treat a variety of conditions ranging from simple dry eyes to complex conditions like glaucoma.

- Visine, for instance, reduces eye redness because it contains potassium chloride and tetrahydrozoline hydrochloride, a vasoconstrictor to constrict or tighten small, superficial blood vessels of the eye, making them small enough you can no longer see them, making the "red" disappear.
- Eye infections can be treated with combinations of corticosteroids and antibiotics in a saline solution applied to the eye. For example, TobraDex is commonly prescribed to patients following cataract surgery to reduce inflammation and prevent infection. It contains tobramycin (an antibiotic) and dexamethasone (a corticosteroid).
- Conjunctivitis, or pink eye, primarily afflicts children and can be caused by viruses, bacteria, allergies, or chemicals. Conjunctivitis literally means *inflammation of the conjunctiva,* and makes the eye appear red, goopy, crusty, and swollen. It is highly contagious. If a virus causes it, there is little that drugs can do to treat it. When it has a bacterial cause, however, it is treated topically with an antibiotic. A couple of common topical antibiotics are bacitracin eye ointment (a generic drug) and AK-Spore (a brand name drug).
- Drugs like Patanol can be administered for treatment of allergic symptoms (itchy, red, watery eyes); others are used to dilate the eyes, like the drug Mydriacyl, or to treat glaucoma, like the drug Diamox. It should be noted that some ophthalmic medications affect the body systemically to some extent, like some used in conjunction with glaucoma.

Matching.
Match the medication to its administration route.

1. ___ Patanol
2. ___ Visine
3. ___ antibiotics
4. ___ TobraDex
5. ___ Diamox
6. ___ dexamethasone
7. ___ carbamide peroxide
8. ___ Mydriacyl
9. ___ tobramycin
10. ___ corticosteroids

A. otic
B. ophthalmic
C. both

TOPICAL – DENTAL AND INHALATION

Dental

Most drugs for dental issues have a local effect. Local anesthetics deaden the nerves in and around the teeth and can be applied via a swish, a spray, or a gel. A variety of different drugs may be used, including **lidocaine** (Xylocaine), **articaine/epinepherine** (Septocaine), **mepivacaine** (Carbocaine), **prilocaine** (Citanest), and **bupivacaine** (Marcaine).

Tooth whitening has become very popular in recent years. **Carbamide peroxide** gel is applied directly to the teeth, making them become whiter and brighter. (Interestingly, carbamide peroxide is the same medication applied to the ear canal for wax buildup.)

Inhalation

Inhalation administration involves the taking in of air, or of breathing in a drug, which then either affects the airway and lungs directly, or is absorbed through the lungs for a systemic effect. **Albuterol** dilates the bronchi on contact, easing breathing in an asthma attack, and is an example of a drug with a local effect; **Imitrex inhaler**, used to treat migraines, is an example of an inhaled drug with a systemic effect.

Realistically, this route is simply referred to as inhalational; if the resulting location effect is important to the report it's clarified as local or systemic.

Also used to target the symptoms of asthma is a device called a **nebulizer**. This takes the liquid form of a medicine and pumps oxygen through it, turning it into a vapor, which is more easily assimilated into the lungs to provide faster relief.

True/False.
Mark the following true or false.

1. Most drugs for dental administration don't have a local effect.

    ○ true

    ○ false

2. A common use for inhalers is to treat asthma.

    ○ true

    ○ false

3. Carbamide peroxide can be applied to the teeth to whiten them.

    ○ true

    ○ false

4. Inhalational application of medication can have a local or systemic effect.

    ○ true

    ○ false

Spelling.
Determine if the following words are spelled correctly. If the spelling is correct, leave the word as it has already been entered. If the spelling is incorrect, retype the word with the correct spelling. Pay particular attention to capitalization.

1. lidocaine _____

2. sitenest _____

3. carbomid paraxide _____

4. enhilation _____

5. Xylocane _____

TOPICAL – SKIN AND NOSE

Skin

This involves using the skin as an administration route. This route usually involves applying medication to a specific area of the skin, or to a wound, to anesthetize it, clean it, or otherwise aid in healing.

Typically you think of the skin as synonymous with **topical**. Certainly, it is one of the primary drug administration routes and is used for a variety of different medications, including many available over-the-counter:

- Lotions and emollients to hydrate the skin and make it soft.
- Antibiotic ointments like **Neosporin**, which is in almost every first aid kit.
- Astringents such as **Calamine** lotion draw together tissues, protect the skin, and help to stop bleeding.
- Antifungals such as miconazole used to treat athlete's foot and **Lamisil** for "jock itch."
- Cleansers such as **Betadine** for cleaning out wounds.
- Premedicated pads such as Tucks for the treatment of hemorrhoids.
- Sprays like **Dermoplast** and **benzocaine**, which relieve pain.
- Antivirals like **Abreva** to treat cold sores.

Intranasal

This involves using the inside of the nose as an administration route. For the purposes of topical drug administration, the use of the intranasal route would be primarily to deal with medical problems related to the nose, such as nosebleeds, and provide medication to areas reachable by nose, such as the sinuses, to relieve congestion and swelling. This method includes such medications as **Flonase**, **Nasonex**, and **Afrin**.

Matching.
Match the drug to its administration route.

1. ____	emollients	A.	skin
2. ____	Afrin	B.	nose
3. ____	Betadine		
4. ____	Dermoplast		
5. ____	Nasonex		

TOPICAL – VAGINAL

Vaginal

The final topical administration route we will cover is the vagina. Several drugs may be inserted into the vagina for treatment of issues related to that local area.

- Vaginal drugs are generally in the form of a cream or suppository. Examples of antifungal suppositories used to treat vaginal infections are **Gyne-Lotrimin**, **Monistat**, and **Vagistat**. Symptoms of vaginal infections are also treated topically with powders, creams, or sprays.
- A **spermicide** can be in a cream or suppository form, inserted into the vagina to kill sperm and prevent pregnancy.

Some drugs administered vaginally can have a systemic effect. For example, a common treatment for low levels of the female hormone **progesterone** is a vaginal suppository, inserted into the vagina where it is assimilated into the soft tissues and then the bloodstream, raising the level of progesterone in the body.

True/False.
Mark the following true or false.

1. Vaginal infections can be treated by either a cream or a suppository.
    - ○ true
    - ○ false

2. Vagistat is administered orally.
    - ○ true
    - ○ false

3. Most drugs administered vaginally have a local effect.
    - ○ true
    - ○ false

4. Drugs administered vaginally cannot have a systemic effect.
    - ○ true
    - ○ false

REVIEW: TOPICAL

Matching.
Match the appropriate terms below.

1. ____ vaginal
2. ____ otic
3. ____ ophthalmic
4. ____ inhalation
5. ____ vasoconstrictor

A. breathed in
B. inside the eye
C. inserted into the vagina
D. pertaining to the ear
E. tightens blood vessels

Spelling.
Determine if the following words are spelled correctly. If the spelling is correct, leave the word as it has already been entered. If the spelling is incorrect, retype the word with the correct spelling. Pay special attention to capitalization.

1. corticosteriods _____

2. Monistat _____

3. Neosporin _____

4. Aphran _____

5. benzocaine _____

6. albuterol _____

7. Todradexx _____

8. potassium chloride _____

9. Mydracile _____

ENTERAL METHODS

Enteral means relating to or inside the intestines. Drugs administered enterally have an intended systemic effect. This is by far the most common way that drugs are administered. Usually, they are taken orally.

The moment that you put a drug into your mouth, it begins to be absorbed: first in the mouth, then in the stomach. From there, most of the drug passes through the intestinal wall and through the liver. This process both chemically alters the drug and dilutes it before it ever makes its way into your bloodstream. Many factors determine how much that drug is affected. How much and what types of food are in your stomach? How effective is your liver? How much of the drug will be diluted or changed before it reaches your bloodstream?

These factors are the reasons that some drugs should be taken on an empty stomach and others should only be taken with food. Still others cannot be effective taken orally at all and are administered via a different (parenteral or topical) route.

Other factors, such as the patient's state of consciousness, the emergent or life-saving nature of the medication, or other problems with the gastrointestinal system can require another route (besides the mouth) be used. However, it is still considered an enteral administration route if that other method uses the gastrointestinal system.

A gastroduodenal feeding tube is an example of enteral administration that bypasses the mouth. A few different types of feeding tubes include:

nasogastric tube: Also called an NG tube, this is passed through the nose, down the esophagus, and into the stomach.

G-tube: A gastric or a **gastrostomy** feeding tube, this is inserted via a small incision directly into the stomach. A similar tube, also inserted (usually via laparoscopy) for feeding is a percutaneous endoscopic gastrostomy (or PEG) tube.

jejunostomy tube: This is smaller than a gastric tube and, as you might suspect, is inserted into the jejunum instead of the stomach.

Drugs can also be administered **rectally** by either suppository or an enema. Since this uses the gastrointestinal tract (albeit the other end) it falls into the category of enteral administration. Most drugs administered via the rectum have a systemic effect and are generally in the form of a suppository. A **suppository** is a small plug or cone of medicine inserted in a body cavity other than the mouth (specifically the rectum or the vagina) and designed to melt at body temperature, being absorbed into the surrounding soft mucosa. They are considered enteral because they are assimilated through the digestive tract. An example is a glycerin or bisacodyl suppository to treat constipation. A common trade name example of this drug is **Dulcolax**.

Terminology.
Enter each term in the space provided. Read the definition and description for each term.

1. nasogastric tube _____

Tube passing from the nose to the stomach.

2. suppository _____

Small plug or cone of medicine inserted in a body cavity other than the mouth.

3. PEG _____

Percutaneous endoscopic gastrostomy.

4. gastrostomy _____

Surgical opening of the stomach.

5. G-tube _____

Gastric feeding tube.

Multiple Choice.
Choose the best answer.

1. The most common drug administration route is _____.

   ○ topical

   ○ enteral

   ○ parenteral

2. The most common enteral route is _____.

   ○ oral

   ○ gastric

   ○ rectal

3. The trade name suppository for treating constipation is spelled _____.

   ○ Dulcolax

   ○ dulcolax

   ○ Dulcalax

   ○ dulcolex

4. The generic name for a suppository for treating constipation is _____.

   ○ Bisacodyl

   ○ bisacodyl

   ○ strenuoius

   ○ strenuous

5. A common ingredient in suppositories to treat constipation is _____.

   ○ glycerine

   ○ glycerin

   ○ Glycerin

   ○ Glycerine

ENTERAL FORMS

Enteral medications are assimilated into the body through the gastrointestinal system, and the primary method for getting them into the body is through the mouth. Drugs come in many different forms and these forms are absorbed differently by the body.

Oral medications can be either solids or liquids. Examples of each include:

Solids	Liquids
powders	syrups
capsules	elixirs
tablets	gels
pills	tinctures
caplets	suspensions
lozenges	

The difference between them is a difference in form, shape, coating, and sometimes it's just a difference in the name. After all, a tablet and a pill are different words for the exact same thing and the terms are used interchangeably.

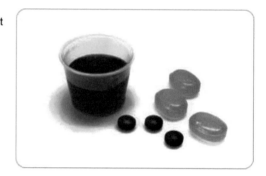

Medications can be specifically formulated to act immediately upon entering the body or they can release more slowly over a period of time. Compared to other types of drugs, these are made to take a long time to be assimilated by the body. This is generally reflected in the name of the medication itself and is often abbreviated. All of the terms listed below mean pretty much the same thing but will appear as part of the name in brand name drugs, so they need to appear in the medical report exactly as they are written/dictated. Some of these are:

- long-acting (LA)
- sustained-release (SR)
- extended-release (ER)
- controlled-release (CR)
- extended-release (XL)

There are many examples of medications that are formulated this way. Some of these are included in the exercise below. Many of the drugs listed (as well as most others with an extended-release form) have another form of the same drug that is not extended, prolonged, or delayed release. Often called "immediate release" in reference, the abbreviation IR is rarely included in the brand name.

Enter Abbreviations.
Enter the abbreviation and what it stands for.

CR: controlled-release
Nalex CR – A cold medicine

1. _____ (Abbreviation)
2. _____

ER: extended-release
Depakote ER – An anticonvulsant and a mood-stabilizing drug

3. _____ (Abbreviation)
4. _____

LA: long-acting
Inderal LA – A beta blocker

5. _____ (Abbreviation)
6. _____

XL: extended-release
Glucotrol XL – An antidiabetic

7. _____ (Abbreviation)
8. _____

SR: sustained-release
Wellbutrin SR – An antidepressant

   9. _____ (Abbreviation)

   10. _____

PARENTERAL – IN THE MOUTH

The mouth is still one of the easiest and least invasive routes of drug administration. There are a couple of different ways that drugs can be administered using the mouth, and that doesn't even count swallowing a pill (remember that is enteral administration). This method includes the area inside of the cheek and under the tongue. The area underneath the tongue is more **permeable** (capable of being penetrated, particularly by a liquid or a gas) and has a rich blood supply, which means that substances can be assimilated very quickly from here. However, it also is constantly being "washed out" with saliva, which makes it harder to administer drugs that require longer-term placement. On the other hand, the inside of the cheek has a nice, big area of smooth muscle that allows for sustained delivery applications and is less permeable, meaning it takes longer for the body to absorb the medication. Depending on the end result, either one could be more or less desirable.

Buccal

This refers to the area inside the cheek. The drug is placed between the upper gums and the cheek. Traditionally, this has been in the form of a patch, but in recent years, tablets have been developed for buccal mucosa delivery. More than one type of drug can be administered this way. In fact, several different drugs with totally different purposes can be assimilated by the body through the buccal mucosa. A few of these include:

Nicotine gum:Delivers doses of nicotine to the blood-vessel-rich areas of the mouth. This drug is used in smoking cessation programs to administer measurably smaller and smaller doses of nicotine to the patient, with the intent to wean them from nicotine completely. NicoDerm CQ and Habitrol are brand-name nicotine gum products.

Testosterone:A male hormone, used to treat testosterone deficiency in men. Marketed as Striant.

Sublingual

This refers to the area under the tongue. Surprisingly, this can be one of the fastest ways for a drug to get into your system. It bypasses the gastrointestinal system, and it is both assimilated quicker and causes less breakdown or change in the chemistry of the drug itself. This is facilitated because lots of blood vessels are located under the tongue.

buprenorphine SL:An opioid, ironically used for treatment of opioid dependence. A patient is given sublingual doses of narcotic buprenorphine, under a brand name such as **Subutex**, in order to avoid severe withdrawal symptoms.

nitroglycerin SL:A vasodilator that relaxes blood vessels, easing the workload of the heart.

isosorbide dinitrate SL:A vasodilator used to dilate the blood vessels, which helps to both prevent and alleviate heart pain.

Matching.
Match the correct term to the definition.

1. ____ sublingual
2. ____ permeable
3. ____ buprenorphine
4. ____ nitroglycerin SL
5. ____ buccal

A. in the cheek
B. can be penetrated
C. relaxes blood vessels
D. a narcotic
E. under the tongue

Multiple Choice.
Choose the best answer.

1. The patient was instructed to place the tablet under the lip, just above the teeth. This is an example of _____ administration.

   ○ buccal

   ○ sublingual

2. It is possible for the tongue and cheek to be used as drug administration routes because the mucosa is _____.

   ○ dilated

   ○ permeable

   ○ in the mouth

3. A brand name drug used to treat opioid dependence is _____.

   ○ Subutex

   ○ buprenorphine SL

4. A generic drug used to treat opioid dependence is _____.

   ○ Subutex

   ○ buprenorphine SL

5. A spray administered under the tongue to alleviate angina-related pain is an example of a _____ administration.

   ○ buccal

   ○ sublingual

6. Dilating the blood vessels can treat symptoms of angina, or chest pain. A generic drug that does this is _____.

   ○ isosorbide dinitrate SL

   ○ Isosordil

PARENTERAL – BREATHING IT IN

Parenteral drugs can be administered by breathing them in. Most inhaled drugs have a systemic effect; however, some, like rescue inhalers for the treatment of asthma, have an intended local effect. This is accomplished through either of the ways that people breathe—through the mouth or the nose.

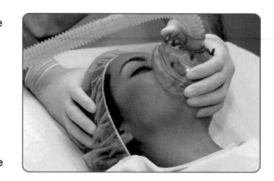

Inhalational

The most common medication administered via inhalation with a systemic effect is anesthesia, used both to begin and to maintain a **general anesthesia**. General anesthesia is for pain control, often during surgery, and is characterized by unconsciousness, muscle relaxation, and a total loss of sensation throughout the entire body. It is administered using either a face mask or an endotracheal tube. An **endotracheal tube** is a catheter inserted into the patient's trachea to provide or maintain an airway. Only **anesthesiologists** administer general anesthesia drugs.

nitrous oxide:Also called laughing gas. This anesthetic relieves pain and causes relaxation and forgetfulness but usually without putting a patient under.

desflurane:A potent inhalational anesthetic that is used during surgery to accomplish general anesthesia. Its brand name is **Suprane**.

True/False.
Mark the following true or false.

1. General anesthesia can be administered through a face mask or endotracheal tube.

    ○ true

    ○ false

2. Nitrous oxide is also known as laughing gas.

    ○ true

    ○ false

PARENTERAL – INTRAVENOUS INJECTIONS

A needle injection—it makes a lot of people squeamish. Fortunately, there's just one way to do that, right? Wrong! Actually, there are a number of ways to "inject" medicine into a patient. Of all the different routes used to administer drugs parenterally, a needle is the most common. The size and type of needle, as well as where it is injected, determine what specific type of parenteral administration route is being used.

The term **gauge** describes the size of a needle. Basically, the smaller the number the larger the diameter of the needle. A 20-gauge needle is larger in diameter than a 30-gauge needle and is the most common gauge size used in hospitals to give intravenous injections. A 30-gauge needle is considered fairly small in diameter and is the size often used by patients to give themselves subcutaneous insulin injections. When you donate blood, the phlebotomist will most likely use a large gauge needle, a size 16 or 18—ouch!

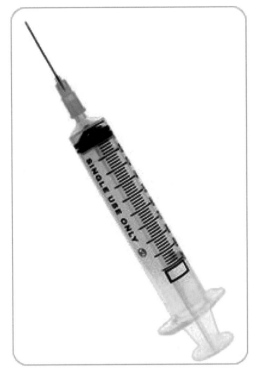

Intravenous

Intravenous involves injecting medication directly into a vein using a needle and syringe. As with other parenteral types of administration, the drugs bypass the gastrointestinal system, thereby avoiding both the delay of effect and the chemical alteration that can occur. In its simplest form, a **syringe** containing the drug is attached to a hollow needle, and the drug is injected directly into a vein, generally a vein in the arm. A syringe is pictured here.

- Within the walls of the hospital, other methods of administering the drugs are even more common. A **peripheral IV line** consists of a short catheter inserted into any vein that is not in the chest or abdomen. It's usually a hand or arm vein, although veins of the legs and feet, neck, and (with babies) the scalp can also be used. This catheter creates a nice portal into the body, and a syringe or other type of IV system can quickly and easily be hooked up to it and drugs can be administered.

Matching.
Match the correct term to the definition.

1. ____ IV
2. ____ gauge
3. ____ syringe

A. a small device for injecting fluids
B. intravenous
C. needle diameter

Multiple Choice.
Choose the best answer.

1. Of the following, which needle gauge represents the smallest diameter of needle?

   ○ 14 gauge

   ○ 18 gauge

   ○ 22 gauge

PARENTERAL – STILL INJECTING IT

Intravenous (cont.)

- **Central IV line** or a **central venous catheter** – Another portal for administrating intravenous drugs. Much like with a peripheral IV line, a catheter is inserted for quick, easy drug administration. The difference is that the central venous catheter is placed into a large vein, the superior or inferior vena cava, or even within the atrium of the heart itself. Because the medication is added to a large, rapidly flowing vein, it does not burn as much when it's added (some medications, like vancomycin, are caustic and can cause phlebitis). This is an advantage of a central line. A central line can be inserted through what is called a **PICC** or peripherally inserted central catheter. The line is inserted through a vein in the arm and threaded upwards until it is in the superior vena cava or right atrium. This is often necessary when a patient will require intravenous access for a long time.

- **Total parenteral nutrition** – Typically administered via a central line. With TPN 100% of the patient's nutrition is received via an intravenous line, eliminating the need for both eating and digesting. The "nutrition" is a liquid containing various amino acids, lipids, vitamins, salts, and glucose. This is necessary when a patient has undergone major surgery and their digestive system cannot properly function, or when a patient is in a coma or otherwise unconscious and requires nutrition.

- In addition to nutritional fluid, virtually any other kind of medication can be administered intravenously. In the hospital, it is fast and easy to administer, quick and sure in its effect. Drugs are administered intravenously in several ways:

intravenous drip: This is the continuous infusion of fluid (which can be accomplished with or without medication) through any of the IV access devices. The drug is administered slowly over time.

bolus: The administration of medication in a single, large dose. The drug is administered all at once.

piggyback: Intermittent infusion. This typically involves a smaller IV bag added into the existing IV line to administer doses of medication.

Matching.
Match the correct term to the definition.

1. ____ bolus   A. peripherally inserted central catheter

2. ____ PICC   B. total parenteral nutrition

3. ____ TPN   C. single, large dose

Multiple Choice.
Choose the best answer.

1. A drug administered slowly over time.

   ○ intravenous drip

   ○ bolus

2. A drug administered all at once.

   ○ intravenous drip

   ○ bolus

3. Which of the following is NOT a portal for the administration of intravenous drugs.

   ○ PICC

   ○ total parenteral nutrition

   ○ peripheral IV line

   ○ central venous line

4. A _____ has the advantage of injecting the drug directly into the heart.

   ○ syringe

   ○ peripheral IV line

   ○ central IV line

5. A _____ is inserted into a peripheral vein and then threaded to the superior vena cava or right atrium.

   ○ syringe

   ○ PICC

   ○ central venous line

PARENTERAL – OTHER WAYS

Intramuscular or IM

This utilizes a long needle with a large diameter. A large, long needle is needed in order to get through all the layers on top of your muscle because the needle reaches all the way inside a muscle to deliver its contents. Generally large muscles of the body are the best: hips, gluteals, and large muscles of the legs. Babies and kindergarteners receive their vaccinations IM. Many different types of other drugs can also be administered IM, including antibiotics, follicle-stimulating hormones, and hCG as protocol for in vitro fertilization.

Subcutaneous

A short, small diameter needle is used to inject medication through the skin. It is much easier to get to the layer of fat directly under the skin than all the way into a vein or a muscle. Subcutaneous is often abbreviated in medical reports as **subcu**, **subq**, or **SQ**. Insulin required by insulin-dependent diabetics is injected subcutaneously with a systemic effect. Novocain injections for dental procedures are also administered subcutaneously, but have a local effect.

Spinal

The spinal administration route is accomplished with a needle injected directly into the spinal canal. This can achieve a different result dependent upon where in the spinal canal it is inserted.

- A spinal block is delivered directly into the spinal fluid, and is a one-time injection. This can be used for pain control during and after a caesarean section.
- An epidural is delivered into the epidural space surrounding the spine, and is designed to deliver continuous pain relief. Epidurals are often used during childbirth.

Multiple Choice.
Choose the best answer.

1. Subcu or subq are both acceptable ways to represent what type of administration route?
   - ○ intramuscular
   - ○ intravenous
   - ○ subcutaneous

2. Refers to a needle injection directly into a muscle.
   - ○ intramuscular
   - ○ intravenous
   - ○ subcutaneous

3. Refers to a needle injection directly into a vein.
   - ○ intramuscular
   - ○ intravenous
   - ○ subcutaneous

4. Requires a short needle, small in diameter.
   - ○ intramuscular
   - ○ intravenous
   - ○ subcutaneous

5. Requires a long needle, large in diameter.
   - ○ intramuscular
   - ○ intravenous
   - ○ subcutaneous

REVIEW: ENTERAL AND PARENTERAL

True/False.
Mark the following true or false.

1. Enteral means relating to or inside the intestines.

    ○ true

    ○ false

2. When used with medications, the abbreviation LA stands for long-acting.

    ○ true

    ○ false

3. Sublingual refers to the area inside the cheek.

    ○ true

    ○ false

4. The most common drug administration route is parenteral.

    ○ true

    ○ false

Matching.
Match the correct term to the definition.

1. ____ tube passing from the nose to the stomach	A.	inhalational
2. ____ drugs administered through the mouth or nose, being breathed into the body	B.	under the skin
	C.	nasogastric
3. ____ injected in the vein	D.	in the muscle
4. ____ bolus	E.	intravenous
5. ____ surgical insertion of a gastric feeding tube	F.	spinal injection
6. ____ intramuscular	G.	gastrostomy
7. ____ subcutaneous	H.	single, large dose
8. ____ epidural		

UNIT 4

Drug Categories

DRUG CATEGORIES – INTRODUCTION

To review, medications are given for one of three main purposes:

- to relieve
- to cure
- to control

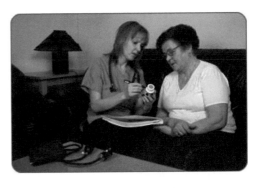

For having only three primary purposes, there are a tremendous amount of unique medical issues that drugs can treat and almost as many drugs to treat them. Some of these we have touched upon: drugs fight bacteria, dilate arteries, and alleviate pain. Drugs can be categorized in a couple different ways. It is not uncommon to categorize them according to body system. What drugs are used to treat issues related to the cardiovascular system? Which ones affect the central nervous system? What drugs address problems in the endocrine system? Of course, the reality is that many drugs can be used to treat problems across a variety of different body systems. In this unit, you will be introduced to a number of different drug categories with medications being lumped together according to what specific function they perform in the body. Of course, all drugs and even all drug categories are not represented in this unit. And in practical application, drugs don't fit into simple nice little categories all that well. More often than not, a prescribed medication will contain more than one kind of drug: for example, the combination of corticosteroids and antibiotics discussed in an earlier unit. An understanding of these general categories and how they work will be useful as you begin transcription editing and need to glean meaning from content. Regardless of how they are categorized, these are all terms that will come up in actual medical records.

By way of warning, it is a lot of information. True, all of the categories, as well as many of the medications, you will see daily in your work as a medical transcription editor. Even so, it is a lot of information.

The biggest question before you, as a medical transcription editor, is "what do I need to know about drugs to be a great MTE?" In spite of everything that you have learned thus far, you will never be required to diagnose a patient and determine a medication regimen to treat his or her specific problem. You will never administer that medication. You will never write a prescription. You will never be required to cross-reference and understand how different drugs will interact with each other. And fortunately, you will never have to follow up with the patient and be certain that your prescribed treatment was appropriate and actually solved their problem.

> Although drugs can be categorized in many ways, for our purposes we will be categorizing them by the function they perform in the body.

The reality is that drugs will appear in virtually every medical record that you ever edit. Each drug will need to be spelled correctly. If dosage information is given, it must be formatted and represented correctly. And if you know just a little bit about the drug and what it does, or can easily find that information, you will be well on your way to being not just an average MTE, but a great one.

That having been said, there is a LOT of information in this unit. Please don't be overwhelmed by it. You should be able to recognize (and spell) the different drug categories, as well as recognize some of the more common medications that comprise them. There will always be more to learn when it comes to pharmacology! So, read the information, do all the exercises, and you will be surprised at how much you will know when you finish this unit.

DRUG CATEGORIES OVERVIEW

This Drug Categories unit is by far the largest unit in this Pharmacology module, maybe even in the whole training program. It makes sense, of course, for this to be a sizeable unit as there are so many pharmaceuticals used in the medical industry (with more being developed daily). This is not an exhaustive list by any stretch of the imagination, but it is a comprehensive list designed to give you broad exposure to a lot of drugs and their usages.

The categories covered in this unit include:

Cardiovascular Drugs

- Antiarrhythmics
- Anticoagulants
- Antihyperlipidemics
- Antihypertensives
- Vasodilators
- Beta Blockers
- Calcium Channel Blockers

Digestive Drugs

- Antacids
- Antiemetics

Endocrine Drugs

- Diuretics
- Diabetic Medications
- Insulin
- Hormones
- Thyroid Hormones
- Sex Hormones
- Pregnancy and Hormones
- Infertility and Hormones

Immune Drugs

- Antibiotics
- Antivirals
- Antihistamines
- Cytotoxics

Pain Management

- Non-Narcotic Analgesics
- NSAIDs
- Narcotic Analgesics
- Anesthesia
- Corticosteroids

Psychological Drugs

- Antianxiety
- Antidepressants
- Antipsychotics

Respiratory Drugs

- Antihistamines
- Bronchodilators
- Cough Suppressants and Expectorants
- Decongestants

This unit, like other units and modules in this training program, is loaded with exercises, practice, and games to help you absorb the information. It makes great sense to incorporate the drugs you are exposed to in this unit into your word list. A word list, as the name implies, is a list of words collected for quick reference. You will be amazed at how handy word lists can be in medical transcription editing.

CARDIOVASCULAR DRUGS

Cardiovascular drugs are those that affect the function of the heart and blood vessels and are among the most widely used drugs in medicine. As you might imagine, there are a lot of categories that fall under the cardiovascular drug umbrella. For our purposes, we will cover the following:

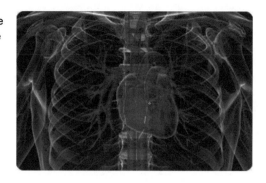

- Antiarrhythmics
- Anticoagulants
- Antihyperlipidemics
- Vasodilators
- Beta Blockers
- Calcium Channel Blockers

Without further ado, we start with the heart!

ANTIARRHYTHMICS

Drugs used to control irregular heartbeats are called **antiarrhythmics**. Normally, the heart beats in a smooth, normal rhythm. When it doesn't, that condition is called **arrhythmia**. That abnormal rhythm can be too fast or too slow or have some other component that is aberrant, such as skipping beats. In any case, arrhythmia can be the normal baseline heartrate for some people, can be an irritating but basically benign condition, or can be a life-threatening emergency.

Antiarrhythmics that either prevent or treat arrhythmia work by changing the nerve impulses in the heart. They can stimulate the involuntary muscles to speed up the heartbeat. They can block those same muscles to reduce the heart rate, or simply reduce the force of the heart muscle contraction. This also lowers blood pressure and can help with chest pain.

Antiarrhythmics include a number of drugs. Following are a couple of generic drugs with their most common brand names:

Generic Name	Trade Name
procainamide	Procan SR and Pronestyl
digoxin	Lanoxin

Lopressor (metoprolol) is also used to treat arrhythmia but falls into a class of drugs called beta blockers that we will learn about shortly.

As an MTE, you will see the following generic drugs frequently. Although these generic drugs also have brand names, they are less commonly seen in medical reports.

- disopyramide
- mexiletine
- amiodarone

True/False.
Mark the following true or false.

1. Antiarrhythmics are a class of drugs that control irregular heartbeats.

   ○ true

   ○ false

2. The generic form of Lopressor is metoprolol.

   ○ true

   ○ false

3. Any arrhythmia is a problem and must be corrected with drugs or surgery.

   ○ true

   ○ false

4. Antiarrhythmics can reduce angina. (Hint: If you're not sure, look up the definition for "angina.")

   ○ true

   ○ false

5. Dysopiramide is the correct spelling for a generic antiarrhythmic.

   ○ true

   ○ false

Multiple Choice.
Choose the correctly spelled term.

1. A generic name of an antiarrhythmic drug.
   - ○ metaprolol
   - ○ metoprolal
   - ○ metoprolol
   - ○ metopralol

2. A generic name of an antiarrhythmic drug.
   - ○ amiodarone
   - ○ amioderone
   - ○ amiodaron
   - ○ amioderon

3. A generic name of an antiarrhythmic drug.
   - ○ procainimide
   - ○ procanimide
   - ○ procanamide
   - ○ procainamide

4. A generic name of an antiarrhythmic drug.
   - ○ disopyramide
   - ○ disopryamide
   - ○ disopyrimide
   - ○ disopryimide

5. A brand name of the antiarrhythmic drug procainamide.
   - ○ procan SR
   - ○ Procan SR
   - ○ Procain SR
   - ○ Procaine SR

6. A generic name of an antiarrhythmic drug.
   - ○ mexilitine
   - ○ mexelitine
   - ○ mexiletine
   - ○ mexeletine

7. A brand name of the antiarrhythmic drug metoprolol.
   - ○ Lopresor
   - ○ Lopressor
   - ○ lopressor
   - ○ lopresor

8. A brand name of the antiarrhythmic drug procainamide.
   - ○ pronestyl
   - ○ Pronestyl
   - ○ pronestil
   - ○ Pronestil

ANTICOAGULANTS

Coagulation is a process whereby liquid blood forms into solid clots. You have probably seen blood clots on a number of occasions in your life. Have you ever had a bloody nose? What happens after it has bled for a while? Have you ever thought about why the body does this? What would happen if the blood did not clot? The slightest wound (or even a bloody nose) could cause a person to bleed to death. Platelets and fibrin immediately begin to surround a damaged blood vessel, forming a clot to both stop the bleeding and begin to repair the vessel.

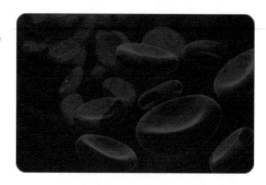

Sometimes, though, a clot can develop inside an artery that completely blocks the flow of blood. This is called thrombosis. This can happen because of trauma, infection, or even due to long periods of being sedentary (such as sitting on a plane for several hours). In any case, clots that appear and completely obstruct the flow of blood are bad. When blood vessels to the brain are obstructed, it causes stroke, which can be lethal.

Drugs that treat or prevent inappropriate clotting of the blood can be divided into two separate categories: those that prevent the formation of clots, which are called **anticoagulants** (these are also sometimes called blood thinners), and those that break up, dissolve, and cause clots to disperse, which are called **thrombolytics**. (Thrombolytics can also prevent clots.) Thrombolytics are usually referred to as "clot busters" and are usually only administered through IV in a hospital setting.

Although there are others, two of the most common injectable anticoagulants are **heparin** and **Lovenox**.

The most commonly prescribed oral anticoagulant is **warfarin**, which is marketed under the brand name **Coumadin**.

Spelling.
Determine if the following words are spelled correctly. If the spelling is correct, leave the word as it has already been entered. If the spelling is incorrect, retype the word with the correct spelling.

1. anticoagulent _____

2. warfaran _____

3. heparin _____

4. thrombolityc _____

5. Lovnox _____

Multiple Choice.
Choose the best answer.

1. A common injectable anticoagulant.

    ○ thrombolytic

    ○ heparin

    ○ warfarin

    ○ Coumadin

2. Typically refers to drugs that prevent clotting.

    ○ anticoagulants

    ○ thrombolytics

3. Typically refers to drugs that dissolve and disperse clots.

    ○ anticoagulants

    ○ thrombolytics

4. Brand name for a common anticoagulant.

    ○ Thromboease

    ○ heparin

    ○ warfarin

    ○ Coumadin

5. Brand name for a common injectable anticoagulant.

    ○ Lovenox

    ○ heparin

    ○ warfarin

    ○ Coumadin

ANTIHYPERLIPIDEMICS

Antihyperlipidemics is a big word. Let's take it in pieces, and I bet you already know what types of drugs these are.

Anti-	against, counteracting
hyper-	elevated, above
lipid-	fats
-emics	in the blood

So, what does it mean? Fighting against + too much + fat + in the blood—right? Well, yes, actually. **Hyperlipidemia** is the elevation of lipids in the blood. Primarily this refers to cholesterol (hypercholesterolemia), although it can also mean elevated triglycerides. Everybody knows that too much cholesterol is not a good thing. Why? Why is it bad?

Well, when there is too much cholesterol or other fat in the blood, it can cause hardening of the arteries (atherosclerosis), because the fats deposit plaque on the walls of the arteries. Too much plaque and the blood has a hard time getting through. That can lead to a heart attack. And we know that's bad.

These drugs are also called **lipid-lowering agents**, and they work in a couple of different ways by decreasing the body's production of cholesterol.

There are a few different categories of antihyperlipidemics. First and most common are the **statin** drugs. They are so called because, well, they all end in -statin. It really helps make it easy to identify when they give drugs such similar names, don't you think? They work by slowing down an enzyme that is important in the creation of cholesterol. Here are a few of the common statin drugs:

Generic Name	Trade Name
atorvastatin	Lipitor
lovastatin	Mevacor
simvastatin	Zocor

Another type of antihyperlipidemics is bile acid sequestrants. These are cool. They target the bile acids that contain cholesterol when they enter the gut and prevent them from being reabsorbed back into the gut. This includes **cholestyramine**, which is sold under the brand name **Questran**, and **colestipol**, sold as **Colestid**.

A couple different kinds of antihyperlipidemics work on lowering triglycerides. First is niacin, which is a vitamin also known as vitamin B3. Fibrates are also used to lower triglycerides and include the drugs **gemfibrozil**, sold under the brand name **Lopid**, and **fenofibrate**, which is sold under the brand name **TriCor**.

Matching.
Match the generic drug to its trade name.

1. ___	cholestyramine	A.	Colestid
2. ___	lovastatin	B.	Lipitor
3. ___	fenofibrate	C.	Lopid
4. ___	atorvastatin	D.	Mevacor
5. ___	simvastatin	E.	Questran
6. ___	gemfibrozil	F.	TriCor
7. ___	colestipol	G.	Zocor

Multiple Choice.
Choose the correct spelling of the term.

1. A brand name of an antihyperlipidemic statin drug.

   ○ Mevocor

   ○ Mevacor

   ○ Mevacore

   ○ Mevocore

2. An antihyperlipidemic drug that is used to lower triglycerides.

   ○ fenofibrate

   ○ fenafibrate

   ○ fenofibrat

   ○ fenafibrat

3. A generic name of an antihyperlipidemic statin drug.

   ○ atorovastatin

   ○ atoravastatin

   ○ atorvatatin

   ○ atorvastatin

4. A brand name of an antihyperlipidemic drug that is used to lower triglycerides.

   ○ Lopid

   ○ Lobid

   ○ Lo-Bid

   ○ Lo-Pid

5. The brand name of the antihyperlipidemic drug atorvastatin.

   ○ Lipator

   ○ Lipitor

   ○ Lipitore

   ○ Lipatore

6. A generic antihyperlipidemic that targets the bile acids that contain cholesterol.

   ○ cholestyramin

   ○ colestyramin

   ○ colestyramine

   ○ cholestyramine

7. A generic antihyperlipidemic that targets the bile acids that contain cholesterol.

   ○ colestipol

   ○ cholestipol

   ○ colestipole

   ○ cholestipole

8. A generic name of an antihyperlipidemic statin drug.

   ○ simvostatin

   ○ sinvostatin

   ○ simvastatin

   ○ sinvastatin

9. The generic name of an antihyperlipidemic drug.

   ○ gemfibrozil

   ○ gimfibrozil

   ○ genfibrozil

   ○ ginfibrozil

10. A vitamin that lowers triglycerides.

   ○ niacine

   ○ niocin

   ○ niocine

   ○ niacin

ANTIHYPERTENSIVES

Hypertension refers to an elevation in blood pressure. Although you have heard the term **blood pressure**, have undoubtedly had your own blood pressure taken, and have a general idea what it means, you may find it interesting that blood pressure is technically the force exerted by the circulating blood on the walls of the blood vessels. It is a basic indication of whether there is something wrong in the body. Hypertension can indicate a risk of stroke, heart attack, aneurysm, and even liver failure. If your blood pressure remains elevated for sustained periods of time the pressure of the blood against the vessels literally damages the brain, the eyes, the heart, pretty much anywhere that blood goes.

Drugs that lower blood pressure are called **antihypertensives**. They accomplish this in a couple of different ways, such as interrupting nerve impulses to the brain or causing blood vessels to relax and get bigger. In fact, there are some major classes of medications that are effective antihypertensives. These include **beta blockers**, **calcium channel blockers**, and **diuretics**, all of which will be covered separately later in this unit. In addition to being antihypertensives, these are effective drugs against a number of different problems related to the heart and cardiovascular system.

ACE inhibitors are another class of antihypertensive drugs. They work by stopping a hormone called **angiotensin** from ever forming. This hormone normally causes blood vessels to narrow. A number of ACE inhibitors are routinely prescribed for the treatment of hypertension. They are also useful in treating congestive heart failure. These include:

Generic Name	Trade Name
enalapril	Vasotec
fosinopril	Monopril
lisinopril	Zestril
captopril	Capoten

Other drugs that are commonly used to treat high blood pressure are:

Generic Name	Trade Name
clonidine	Catapres
methyldopa	Aldoril

True/False.
Mark the following true or false.

1. Hypertension means low blood pressure.

   ○ true

   ○ false

2. ACE inhibitors are rarely prescribed for high blood pressure.

   ○ true

   ○ false

3. Hypertension can indicate a higher risk of other diseases, such as heart attack and stroke.

   ○ true

   ○ false

4. ACE inhibitors are useful in treating congestive heart failure.

   ○ true

   ○ false

5. High blood pressure itself can't cause damage.

   ○ true

   ○ false

Matching.
Match the generic drug to its trade name.

1. ____ clonidine

2. ____ fosinopril

3. ____ captopril

4. ____ methyldopa

5. ____ enalapril

6. ____ lisinopril

A. Aldoril

B. Capoten

C. Catapres

D. Monopril

E. Vasotec

F. Zestril

VASODILATORS

The term **vasodilators** is sometimes used interchangeably with antihypertensives and sometimes classified separately. Vasodilators are actually muscle relaxants, but they work directly on the smooth muscles of the blood vessel walls, causing them to widen (or dilate). A primary use is in the treatment of hypertension (thus the classification as antihypertensives), and most vasodilators are prescribed for that purpose.

Hydralazine is a by-the-book vasodilator. It opens up the blood vessels, making it easier for the heart to pump and lowering blood pressure. It is sold under the brand name **Apresoline**. The generic drugs **phentolamine** and **prazosin** both lower blood pressure by relaxing the blood vessels.

A common vasodilator you may have heard of, **minoxidil**, was initially developed to treat high blood pressure. It was quickly discovered to have an interesting side effect: hair growth. Specifically, it was found to be effective at reversing baldness. Enterprising drug companies reformulated it from a pill form to a topical form and have sold millions of them in the United States under the brand name **Rogaine**.

Another vasodilator is **isosorbide**. It is considered a nitrate and works by relaxing blood vessels and allowing blood vessels to dilate. You have already learned that a by-product of dilating the blood vessels is lowering blood pressure. However, isosorbide is prescribed primarily to treat angina or chest pain. Although sold under a number of different brand names, **Imdur** and **Isordil** are common ones.

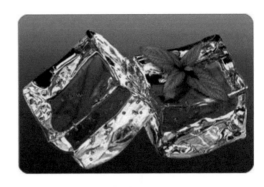

Perhaps the most commonly used vasodilator is **nitroglycerin**. This is sold under different brand names, but especially **Nitro** and **Nitro-Bid**. Like other vasodilators, it relaxes the blood vessels. Although it has the effect of lowering blood pressure, it is more frequently used to treat chest pain, at least chest pain caused by the heart.

Most **angina**—chest pain directly attributed to the heart not getting enough oxygen—can be relieved by opening up the blood vessels, allowing more blood (and hence more oxygen) to get to the heart. **Nitroglycerin** does this quickly and has been doing it for a very long time. It was first used to treat "heart pain" in 1879! Pretty impressive when you consider that poor Joseph Lister was still desperately trying to convince the medical community that it was "gentlemanly" for doctors to wash their hands after performing surgery or tending to the dead and dying! Nitroglycerin is administered sublingually and its effect is very quick.

Listerine was named after Joseph Lister in 1879 because of his ground-breaking work on germs and cleanliness.

Multiple Choice.
Choose the correct spelling of the term.

1. A generic drug that lowers blood pressure by relaxing the blood vessels.

    ○ phentolomine

    ○ phentalomine

    ○ phentalamine

    ○ phentolamine

2. A generic vasodilator that has hair growth as a side effect.

    ○ minoxidil

    ○ menoxidil

    ○ minoxadil

    ○ menoxadil

3. A drug that relaxes the smooth muscle in the blood vessels.

    ○ vasadilators

    ○ vasodilators

    ○ vasadilaters

    ○ vasodilaters

4. A generic vasodilator used to lower blood pressure.
   - ○ prazosin
   - ○ prazocin
   - ○ prasocin
   - ○ prasosin

5. A brand name nitroglycerin.
   - ○ Nitrobid
   - ○ Nitro-Bid
   - ○ nitrobid
   - ○ Nitrobide

6. A generic vasodilator used to lower blood pressure.
   - ○ isasorbide
   - ○ isosarbide
   - ○ isosorbid
   - ○ isosorbide

7. A generic name for a vasodilator.
   - ○ hydralazine
   - ○ hydrolazine
   - ○ hydralozine
   - ○ hydralasine

8. A brand name of the nitrate isosorbide.
   - ○ Indur
   - ○ Imdur
   - ○ Indure
   - ○ Imdure

9. A vasodilator that lowers blood pressure and treats chest pain.
   - ○ nitroglycerine
   - ○ nitroglycerin
   - ○ nitroglyserine
   - ○ nitroglyserin

10. A brand name of the generic vasodilator hydralazine.
    - ○ Apresoline
    - ○ Apressoline
    - ○ Apresolin
    - ○ Apressolin

BETA BLOCKERS

Beta blockers are a class of drugs used frequently in the treatment of cardiac conditions. Basically, they work by blocking the action of adrenaline in your body. Why would you want to block your adrenaline? Because it slows down your heartbeat and makes it beat with less force, helping blood vessels relax and open up. Slower heartbeat, opened-up blood vessels=lower blood pressure, right? Absolutely. Beta blockers are effective at lowering blood pressure.

It turns out that they also do a number of other things to protect and heal the body. First, they help your heart in a number of ways. Beta blockers are used to treat arrhythmia (irregular heart beat), heart failure, chest pain, prevent heart attack, and aid healing following a heart attack.

They are also effective in treating glaucoma, migraines, anxiety disorders, and certain kinds of tremors.

Some beta blockers include:

Generic Name	Trade Name
propranolol	Inderal
atenolol	Tenormin
metoprolol	Lopressor
timolol*	Betimol

*This is used primarily to treat glaucoma

Historically, beta blockers have been contraindicated for congestive heart failure. However, recently (September 2007) one called **carvedilol** has been approved in the United States for treatment of mild to moderate congestive heart failure.

Multiple Choice.
Choose the best answer.

1. Beta blockers do NOT treat ____.
   - ○ migraines
   - ○ all kinds of tremors
   - ○ heart failure
   - ○ chest pain

2. A beta blocker that can treat congestive heart failure is ____.
   - ○ carvedilol
   - ○ propranolol
   - ○ atenolol
   - ○ timolol

3. ____ can treat glaucoma.
   - ○ atenolol
   - ○ metoprolol
   - ○ timolol
   - ○ propranolol

4. Beta blockers work to block the action of ____.
   - ○ prothrombin
   - ○ estrogen
   - ○ calcium
   - ○ adrenaline

5. Beta blockers cause ____.
   - ○ slower heart rate
   - ○ faster heart rate
   - ○ higher blood pressure
   - ○ irregular heart rate

Spelling.
Determine if the following words are spelled correctly. If the spelling is correct, leave the word as it has already been entered. If the spelling is incorrect, retype the word with the correct spelling. Pay special attention to capitalization.

1. Inderol _____

2. metaprolol _____

3. propranalol _____

4. betimlol _____

5. carvedilol _____

CALCIUM CHANNEL BLOCKERS

Calcium channel blockers are a class of drugs that are effective as treatment for hypertension. Although similar, they work a little differently than beta blockers. **Calcium channel blockers** work on certain types of cells, like those found in the muscles of the heart and the smooth muscles of the blood vessel walls. Unlike beta blockers, they don't work by dilating (or relaxing) the blood vessels. They work directly on the heart itself, decreasing the force of contraction of the muscle. They do this by preventing (blocking) calcium from entering the cells. Hence the name calcium channel blockers. Pretty easy to remember, don't you think?

These drugs are used to treat hypertension, atrial fibrillation, angina, migraines, and Raynaud's disease. Common calcium channel blockers include:

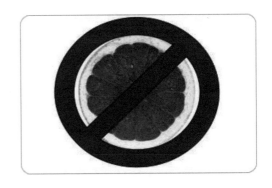

Here is something interesting about calcium channel blockers: they interact with grapefruit. If you eat a grapefruit or drink grapefruit juice while taking a calcium channel blocker, your liver won't be able to eliminate them from your body—causing the medication to continuously build up.

Generic Name	Trade Name
amlodipine	Norvasc
diltiazem	Cardizem
nifedipine	Procardia
verapamil	Calan

True/False.
Mark the following true or false.

1. Calcium channel blockers work directly on the heart.

   ○ true

   ○ false

2. Among other things, calcium channel blockers can treat hypertension, angina, kidney failure, and migraines.

   ○ true

   ○ false

3. The liver is involved in metabolizing calcium channel blockers.

   ○ true

   ○ false

4. Grapefruit and grapefruit juice are not problematic for calcium channel blockers.

   ○ true

   ○ false

5. Blocking calcium causes the heart muscles to contract with more force.

   ○ true

   ○ false

REVIEW: CARDIOVASCULAR DRUGS

Multiple Choice.
Choose the best answer.

1. Beta blockers work by blocking the action of this in the body.
   - ○ heart beat
   - ○ adrenaline
   - ○ headaches
   - ○ oxygen

2. Term for low blood pressure.
   - ○ hypertension
   - ○ hypotension
   - ○ diuretic
   - ○ hypertention

3. ACE inhibitors are in this type of drug class.
   - ○ antihypertensive
   - ○ antihypotensive
   - ○ beta blockers
   - ○ angiotensins

4. Antihyperlipidemics are ___.
   - ○ lipid-elevating agents
   - ○ blood thinners
   - ○ lipid-lowering agents
   - ○ thrombolytics

5. Drugs used to control irregular heartbeats.
   - ○ antiarhythmics
   - ○ arrhythmics
   - ○ arithematics
   - ○ antiarrhythmics

Spelling.
Determine if the following words are spelled correctly. If the spelling is correct, leave the word as it has already been entered. If the spelling is incorrect, retype the word with the correct spelling.

1. metoprolol _____	2. lopresser _____
3. coumadin _____	4. Lipitor _____
5. simvistatin _____	6. mevacor _____
7. warfaran _____	8. Zestryl _____
9. Vasotic _____	10. enalapril _____
11. Isosorbide _____	12. diltizem _____
13. nitrogliceryn _____	14. propranalol _____
15. atenolol _____	

DIGESTIVE DRUGS

There are a variety of medications used to treat digestive problems. Some digestive medications cure digestive problems and others relieve symptoms. The digestive categories we will be covering include:

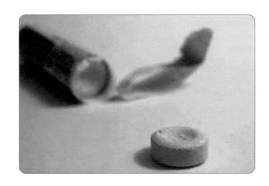

- Antacids
- Antiemetics

Remember, this is not an exhaustive list of digestive medications, simply the basics.

ANTACIDS – LESSON 1

Antacids relieve indigestion and heartburn and sometimes heal ulcers. They work by neutralizing the acid in the stomach. There are a couple of different ways that a drug can do this. First, mineral and salt compounds are a quick and easy way to neutralize stomach acid. These are available without a prescription. A variety of medications are available that utilize three main elements.

1. **Magnesium** – Magnesium is, of course, an element. In fact, it is the 11th most common in the human body. Combined with other elements, as in magnesium carbonate, magnesium trisilicate, and magnesium hydroxide, it is effective in neutralizing stomach acid. Magnesium hydroxide is the most common of these and is known as **milk of magnesia**. Its use can cause diarrhea, so it is also effective at relieving constipation. In this capacity it is referred to as a laxative. You will often see it capitalized because many brand names use it in their name: Phillips' Milk of Magnesia.
2. **Calcium** – Calcium is also an element, and combined in **calcium carbonate** it is a potent and fast-acting antacid. Unlike magnesium hydroxide, calcium carbonate can cause constipation. Calcium also helps to strengthen bones (unless taken to excess). Brand names for calcium carbonate include **Tums** and **Rolaids**.
3. **Aluminum** – Aluminum is a metal element, and when combined into aluminum hydroxide it also is an effective antacid. Brand names include **Amphojel** and **ALternaGEL**. Aluminum hydroxide can cause constipation. It is common to mix it with magnesium hydroxide (which causes diarrhea) to counteract symptoms of constipation. This combination is sold under the brand names **Maalox** and **Mylanta**.

Multiple Choice.
Choose the correctly spelled term.

1. Antacids are used to _____.
   - ○ relieve heartburn
   - ○ relieve indigestion
   - ○ heal ulcers
   - ○ all of the above

2. A(n) _____ is used to treat constipation.
   - ○ laxative
   - ○ antacid
   - ○ calcium carbonate
   - ○ analgesic

3. Of the following, which strengthens bones?
   - ○ magnesium
   - ○ calcium
   - ○ aluminum
   - ○ salts

4. Of the following, which element also works as a laxative?
   - ○ magnesium
   - ○ calcium
   - ○ aluminum
   - ○ salts

5. Which of the following is a brand name for calcium carbonate?
   - ○ Tums
   - ○ magnesium
   - ○ Maalox
   - ○ Mylanta

6. Which of the following is a brand name that combines magnesium and aluminum?

  ○ Tums

  ○ calcium carbonate

  ○ Maalox

  ○ Rolaids

7. A brand name for aluminum hydroxide is spelled _____.

  ○ Alternejel

  ○ Alternajel

  ○ ALternaGEL

  ○ Alternegel

8. The 11th most common element in the human body is spelled _____.

  ○ magnesium

  ○ mangesium

  ○ magnisium

  ○ magniseum

9. The use of _____ can cause constipation.

  ○ magnesium

  ○ Rolaids

  ○ Mylanta

  ○ Maalox

ANTACIDS – LESSON 2

In addition to the compounds covered previously, heartburn, indigestion, and even ulcers can be treated in other ways. H2 blockers and proton pump inhibitors are commonly used. These are also useful in treating gastroesophageal reflux disease (GERD). Many of these are sold by prescription only, although in recent years more have become available over the counter. These are stronger than the mineral and salt combinations discussed above. These are:

H2 blockers – Proteins called histamines encourage acid secretion in the stomach. H2 blockers reduce stomach acid by blocking histamines. In lower dosages, they are available over the counter, although higher dosages require a prescription. These are commonly used for severe heartburn and duodenal ulcers.

Generic Name	Trade Name
famotidine	Pepcid AC
ranitidine	Zantac
nizatidine	Axid
cimetidine	Tagamet

Proton pump inhibitors (PPIs) – These limit stomach acid by shutting down the acid pumps, specifically by blocking an enzyme in the cells themselves. Prescribed and used in treatment of several different kinds of gastric problems, they are especially effective against ulcers.

Generic Name	Trade Name
lansoprazole	Prevacid
omeprazole	Prilosec
esomeprazole	Nexium

There is another drug effective against ulcers that is neither an H2 blocker nor a proton pump inhibitor. Called **sucralfate**, it works by creating a chemical barrier around an ulcer, protecting it, much the way that a Band-Aid protects a wound. A brand name example of this medication is **Carafate**.

Multiple Choice.
Choose the correctly spelled term.

1. A generic name of an H2 blocker.

    ○ nizatadine

    ○ nizatidine

    ○ nizatodine

    ○ nizotidine

2. A drug used to treat ulcers by creating a chemical barrier around the ulcer.

    ○ sucrofate

    ○ sucrafate

    ○ sucrolfate

    ○ sucralfate

3. A generic name of an H2 blocker.

    ○ famotadine

    ○ famotidine

    ○ famortidine

    ○ famotradine

4. A generic name of a proton pump inhibitor.

   ○ lansoprazol

   ○ lansoprazole

   ○ lansoprasole

   ○ lansoprasol

5. A generic name of an H2 blocker.

   ○ simetidine

   ○ cimetadine

   ○ simetadine

   ○ cimetidine

6. A brand name of an H2 blocker antacid.

   ○ Tagamet

   ○ Taggamet

   ○ Tagomet

   ○ tagamet

7. A brand name of a proton pump inhibitor antacid.

   ○ prilosec

   ○ Prilosec

   ○ Prilasec

   ○ prilasec

8. A generic name of an H2 blocker antacid.

   ○ ranitodine

   ○ ranatidine

   ○ Ranitidine

   ○ ranitidine

9. A brand name of an H2 blocker antacid.

   ○ Pepcid AC

   ○ Pepsid AC

   ○ Pepsi AC

   ○ Pepsi Cola

10. A brand name of a proton pump inhibitor antacid.

   ○ Pravesid

   ○ Prevasid

   ○ prevasid

   ○ Prevacid

ANTIEMETICS

Antiemetics are medications that reduce the urge to vomit, also referred to as "antinausea" medications.

How do they work? Well, believe it or not, you actually have a "vomiting center" in your brain and many antiemetics work by blocking messages to that part of your brain. That's why some of these drugs are best taken before you actually need them but when you have a sneaking suspicion that you will. (Think going on an airplane or taking the boat out fishing.)

Other types of antiemetics work by coating the lining of the stomach. These are generally used for motion sickness or following surgery (and specifically the side effects of general anesthesia) or other treatments (such as chemotherapy).

So, what drugs are considered antiemetics? There are several of what we will call the "setron" drugs. We'll call them that because they all end in **-setron**. They include dolasetron, granisetron, ondansetron, tropisetron, and palonosetron. All of these drugs work on that "vomiting center" in the brain and are considered the "gold standard" for treatment of nausea and vomiting due to chemotherapy treatment. So if a drug ends in -setron, you can be pretty sure it's an antiemetic.

Other drugs that work on the brain to relieve nausea and vomiting are the generic drugs **metoclopramide** (sold commonly under the brand name **Reglan**) and **domperidone**. Randomly enough, both of these antiemetics have been found to induce lactation in women as well. The generic drug **scopolamine** is highly effective in the treatment of nausea, vomiting, motion sickness, and intestinal cramping. However, it is also highly toxic and is given only in very small doses. Frighteningly, this is sometimes called the "zombie drug" and is used by criminals to make victims compliant. It completely blocks the formation of any memories whatsoever, literally not allowing the brain to record them. In Colombia, it is referred to as "devil's breath."

Effective antiemetics often can be used for treatment of other conditions. I'm sure that by now you are noticing that this is true of many drugs—putting a powerful agent into your body can have a number of different effects. When you are talking about nausea and vomiting, it is either caused by discomfort of the gastrointestinal system or a signal from the brain. It turns out that the brain is rather important in regulating the entire body, and the gastrointestinal system is the means by which many drugs are taken (think enteral administration).

A few antihistamines are particularly good at controlling symptoms of nausea and vomiting. These include the generic drug **meclizine**, which is the primary ingredient in the over-the-counter brand name **Bonine**. If you have ever lived in a seaside community, you have seen this on the shelf in virtually every store. It is often preferable to the over-the-counter brand name drug **Dramamine** because it does not have as many side effects. Particularly, it does not make one so drowsy that he/she cannot possibly stay awake.

> ## Highlights
>
> Scopolamine, the "devil's breath," has a long history in Colombia. Legend has it that indigenous Colombian tribes used the drug to bury alive the wives and slaves of fallen chiefs so they would quietly accompany their masters into the afterworld.

Also an antihistamine, the generic drug **promethazine** is a more powerful antiemetic. It is commonly sold under the brand name **Phenergan**. In the United States, promethazine is sold by prescription only. However, in the United Kingdom and other countries it is an over-the-counter medication.

Doctors commonly prescribe brand name medications **Compazine** and **Tigan** to treat nausea and vomiting as well.

Finally, **Pepto-Bismol** is considered an antiemetic. This is an over-the-counter medication that treats the symptoms of nausea and vomiting by providing a soothing, protective coat to the lining of the stomach.

Antiemetics are extremely common in medical reports, especially given their prevalence during and after surgery and cancer treatment.

True/False.

Mark the following true or false.

1. All antiemetics work by blocking messages from the vomiting center of the brain.

    ○ true

    ○ false

2. Drugs ending with -setron are antiemetics.

    ○ true

    ○ false

3. Antiemetics are useful in controlling the nausea associated with chemotherapy.

    ○ true

    ○ false

4. Scopolamine has no negative side effects.

    ○ true

    ○ false

5. Antiemetics often have other beneficial effects, such as promoting lactation in women.

    ○ true

    ○ false

6. Dramamine is preferable to Bonine because it does not have drowsiness as a side effect.

    ○ true

    ○ false

7. "Setron" drugs are considered the gold standard for treatment of the side effects of chemotherapy.

    ○ true

    ○ false

8. Domperidone is sometimes called a "zombie" drug.

    ○ true

    ○ false

9. Phenergan is an antihistamine that also acts as an antiemetic, and is available over the counter in the United States.

    ○ true

    ○ false

10. Most antiemetics act on the brain or the gastrointestinal system.

    ○ true

    ○ false

Multiple Choice.
Choose the correct spelling for the term.

1. A generic name for a drug that is highly effective in the treatment of nausea, vomiting, motion sickness, and intestinal cramping.

   ○ scopalomine

   ○ scopolomine

   ○ scopolamine

   ○ scapolomine

2. Medications used to reduce the urge to vomit.

   ○ antimetics

   ○ antimedics

   ○ antiamedics

   ○ antiemetics

3. A brand name of an antiemetic drug.

   ○ Tigan

   ○ Tigane

   ○ Tiagan

   ○ Tiagane

4. An over-the-counter antiemetic that treats symptoms of nausea and vomiting by providing a soothing coat to the stomach's lining.

   ○ Pepto-Bismol

   ○ Pepto-Bismal

   ○ Pepta-Bismal

   ○ Pepta-Bismol

5. A generic antihistamine that is also good at controlling symptoms of nausea and vomiting.

   ○ meclizine

   ○ meclazine

   ○ meclezine

   ○ meclozine

REVIEW: DIGESTIVE DRUGS

Multiple Choice.
Choose the best answer.

1. Antacids work by (○ neutralizing, ○ elevating) acid in the stomach.

2. H2 blockers reduce stomach acid by blocking (○ enzymes, ○ histamines).

3. Tums and Rolaids are brand names for (○ aluminum hydroxide, ○ calcium carbonate).

4. The generic name of Tagamet is (○ cimetidine, ○ famotidine).

5. The medication (○ Tagamet, ○ sucralfate) protects an ulcer by creating a chemical barrier around it.

6. Reglan works on the (○ brain, ○ stomach) to relieve nause and vomiting.

7. Antiemetics work to reduce the urge to (○ vomit, ○ urinate).

8. Setron drugs are considered (○ antacids, ○ antiemetics).

9. The primary ingredient in Bonine is (○ metronidazole, ○ meclizine).

10. The drug (○ Tigan, ○ Tiagan) is a brand name antiemetic.

True/False.

Mark the following true or false.

1. Antacids are available without a prescription.

   ○ true

   ○ false

2. Omeprazole is the generic name of Prevacid.

   ○ true

   ○ false

3. Amphojel is an antacid that includes magnesium.

   ○ true

   ○ false

4. The drug scopolamine is highly toxic and is therefore given in small doses.

   ○ true

   ○ false

5. Some antihistamines are good at controlling symptoms of nausea and vomiting.

   ○ true

   ○ false

6. Pepto-Bismol is considered an antiemetic.

   ○ true

   ○ false

7. Magnesium hydroxide is known to cause diarrhea.

   ○ true

   ○ false

8. Proton pump inhibitors limit stomach acid by shutting down the acid pumps and are especially effective against ulcers.

   ○ true

   ○ false

9. Prilosec is a generic form of a proton pump inhibitor.

   ○ true

   ○ false

10. Promethazine can be purchased in the United States without a prescription.

    ○ true

    ○ false

ENDOCRINE DRUGS

The endocrine system uses blood vessels to regulate or transmit body information. Specifically, glands throughout the body channel hormones into the bloodstream, which then behave as regulators of various body functions. As you might imagine, there are a variety of drug types and conditions that fall under the endocrine drug umbrella. For our purposes, we will cover the following groupings:

- Diuretics
- Hormones
- Diabetes
- Diabetic Medications
- Insulin
- Thyroid Hormones
- Sex Hormones
- Pregnancy and Hormones
- Infertility and Hormones

We begin by diving into diuretics!

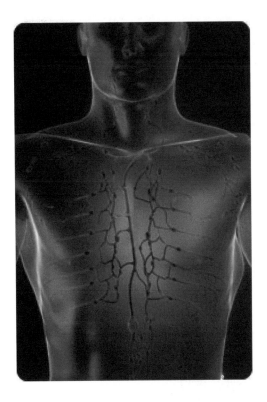

DIURETICS

According to *Dorland's Medical Dictionary*, the word **diuresis** means "increased excretion of urine."* Diuretics, therefore, are drugs that assist the body in getting rid of excess fluid, at the same time increasing the quantity of urine. Most diuretics work on the kidneys, stimulating them to release more sodium. The sodium then takes water out of your blood and tissues. It both eliminates excess fluid and lowers blood pressure, as the subsequent decrease in the amount of fluid reduces the pressure in the arteries. It also gets rid of excess sodium, which is one of the primary reasons for the water retention in the first place.
(*Dorland's Medical Dictionary*, 31st Edition, 2007)

Diuretics get lumped into three or four different categories according to how they actually work on the kidneys. Here are the diuretic drugs that you will likely see often as an MTE.

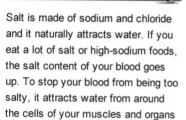

Highlights

Salt is made of sodium and chloride and it naturally attracts water. If you eat a lot of salt or high-sodium foods, the salt content of your blood goes up. To stop your blood from being too salty, it attracts water from around the cells of your muscles and organs to dilute it. This is why salt is blamed both for edema (swelling) and high blood pressure.

Generic Name	Trade Name
hydrochlorothiazide	(sold under a variety of brand names)
furosemide	Lasix
spironolactone	Aldactone

Multiple Choice.
Choose the best answer.

1. Diuretics (⚪ increase, ⚪ decrease) urine output.
2. Sodium in the kidneys helps to (⚪ put water into, ⚪ take water out of) blood and tissues.
3. Diuretics usually work on the (⚪ kidneys, ⚪ liver) .
4. Lasix is the brand name of (⚪ furosemide, ⚪ hydrocholorothiazide) .
5. Eliminating excess fluid in the blood (⚪ increases, ⚪ decreases) blood pressure.

Spelling.
Determine if the following words are spelled correctly. If the spelling is correct, leave the word as it has already been entered. If the spelling is incorrect, retype the word with the correct spelling. Pay special attention to capitalization.

1. hidrochlorathazide _____   2. Lasik _____

3. spironolactone _____   4. aldactone _____

5. Furosomide _____

HORMONES

Of course you are familiar with the term hormones, and you are probably wondering what they are doing as a drug category! Hormones tend to get a bad rap, getting blamed for all kinds of erratic behavior, moodiness, machismo, and minor inconveniences like, say, menopause. But the truth is that hormones are actually a good thing and they are vital to the healthy function of the human body.

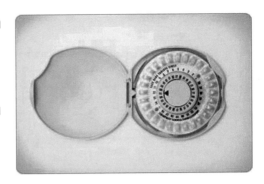

Think of hormones as little messengers. They transmit important messages chemically throughout the body. The word comes from Greek and it means to "impel, urge on." And pretty much, that is just what hormones do. They travel from one cell to another cell or group of cells, "telling" those cells what they need to do to keep things running smoothly. Things like growing, sexual function and reproduction, and mood. They work slowly over time. Produced in the endocrine glands, hormones are powerful chemicals. Just a tiny amount can cause big changes.

So, when do you think hormones are used? Looking at the list of what they are responsible for, can you think of how or why hormones may need to be used as "drugs" in the body?

How about birth control pills? If hormones are responsible for reproduction, what do you suppose is in those little daily pills? Yep—you got it—hormones!

Notice that hormones are also responsible for metabolism. Are there any diseases of metabolism? Before you can appropriately answer that question, you need to be sure that you understand what "metabolism" really means. We often think of it as it relates to food, exercise—things related to losing weight. But it is much, much more than that. According to Cambridge dictionaries, it actually refers to "all the chemical processes in your body." Think things like thyroid function and insulin, puberty, infertility; "all chemical processes" is really quite impressive in scope.

Hormones are responsible for:

- Growth and Development
- Metabolism
- Sexual Function
- Reproduction
- Mood

So, when the messages are not getting sent, or new messages need to be sent, synthetic versions of the hormones are prescribed by doctors, and they are used to assist all of the chemical processes of the body.

DIABETES

Given the propensity towards diabetes in our society, **insulin** is one of the most common and significant hormones used in treatment today. So, what is insulin? It is a hormone secreted by the pancreas; it regulates the glucose (sugar) in the blood. It is essential in converting food into energy. Insulin's counterpart, **glucagon** (also a hormone), stimulates the liver to release stored glucose. The body's inability to produce or properly utilize insulin leads to high levels of sugar (glucose) in the blood and results in a condition called diabetes mellitus, which has reached epidemic proportions in the United States. In the olden days, it used to be called "sugar sickness."

Diabetes can result in all kinds of serious complications. It puts patients at an increased risk for heart disease, stroke, significant damage to the kidneys ultimately causing them to fail, and can lead to blindness—and those are just the major ones. The most common complication of diabetes is called diabetic neuropathy, which refers to the damage caused to nerves throughout the body. Also, foot problems, including poor circulation, swelling, ulcers, and amputation, as well as skin problems can occur.

There are three kinds of diabetes.

Type 1 diabetes: Usually diagnosed in children or young adults. Sometimes called "juvenile diabetes" or "insulin-dependent diabetes mellitus" (IDDM). In type 1 diabetes, the body simply does not produce insulin. It requires life-long administration of insulin.

Type 2 diabetes: Much more common type of diabetes. Sometimes called "noninsulin-dependent diabetes mellitus" (NIDDM) or "adult-onset diabetes mellitus." This type of diabetes generally occurs in patients who are older and have significant risk factors related to lifestyle, specifically poor nutrition, inactivity, and obesity. Unlike type 1 diabetes, the body generally does produce insulin, but it either cannot produce enough or the body cannot use it appropriately. The cells of the body become resistant to the effects of insulin, so more and more insulin is needed in order to do its job.

Gestational diabetes: Of course you know that hormones increase dramatically during pregnancy. These hormonal changes can cause blood sugar elevation resulting in diabetes during the pregnancy. Although it tends to resolve itself after the baby is born, as many as 50% of women who develop gestational diabetes eventually get type 2 diabetes later in life.

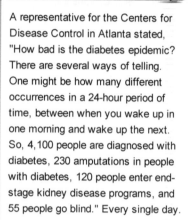

Highlights

A representative for the Centers for Disease Control in Atlanta stated, "How bad is the diabetes epidemic? There are several ways of telling. One might be how many different occurrences in a 24-hour period of time, between when you wake up in one morning and wake up the next. So, 4,100 people are diagnosed with diabetes, 230 amputations in people with diabetes, 120 people enter end-stage kidney disease programs, and 55 people go blind." Every single day.

Matching.
Match the correct term to the definition.

1. ____ type 1 diabetes

2. ____ glucagon

3. ____ gestational diabetes

4. ____ insulin

5. ____ type 2 diabetes

6. ____ diabetes mellitus

A. stimulates the liver to release glucose

B. secreted by the pancreas to regulate glucose

C. juvenile diabetes

D. disease where the body cannot make or use insulin

E. occurs during pregnancy

F. adult-onset diabetes mellitus

Fill in the Blank.
Enter the correct word in the blank provided.

1. Type 1 diabetes mellitus is sometimes called IDDM, which stands for _____.

2. The hormone _____ works to regulate blood sugar.

3. Type 2 diabetes is often referred to as _____ onset diabetes mellitus.

4. Insulin's counterpart, _____, stimulates the liver to release stored glucose.

5. Type 1 diabetes is also called _____ diabetes because of its onset in childhood.

6. Diabetes _____ is the term used to describe the body's inability to make or properly use the hormone insulin.

7. When diabetes occurs only during pregnancy it is called _____ diabetes.

8. Type 2 diabetes is sometimes called NIDDM, which stands for _____.

DIABETIC MEDICATIONS

Now you are aware of how sweeping and serious the problem of diabetes is. You can be absolutely certain you will type it in medical reports. Rarely a day will go by, regardless of what types of reports you typically do, when you will not edit a patient's medical record with diabetes, complications of diabetes, hospital admissions for diabetes, and lots of medications for diabetes. What are those medications? How do you treat diabetes?

Ultimately, the lack of the insulin hormone can best be treated with... brace yourself... insulin! In type 2 diabetes, however, that is the last resort. Patients are strongly encouraged to change their lifestyle, add exercise, closely monitor their blood sugars as well as their sugar intake, and otherwise do whatever they can to avoid having to take insulin. Since insulin is most frequently given as an injection, nobody is excited about having to "shoot" themselves a couple times a day.

One of the first drugs prescribed in the treatment of diabetes is called **metformin**. Not only is it the most commonly prescribed antidiabetic medication, it is one of the most commonly prescribed medications in the United States, period. In 2006 nearly 35,000,000 prescriptions were filled for the generic form of metformin alone! It is sold under the brand name **Glucophage**.

Another antidiabetic medication is **glyburide**. It is sold under the brand names **DiaBeta** and **Micronase**. It works by stimulating the pancreas to produce more insulin. The pancreas has to be capable of producing insulin for glyburide to work, so it cannot be used in type 1 diabetes. Additionally, the brand name drug **Avandia** is used to lower the glucose level in blood.

INSULIN

If diet and exercise have not made a difference and drugs like metformin and glyburide fail to work, or don't work as well, it may become necessary for patients with diabetes to be "put on insulin." Remember the increased risk of stroke and heart disease, circulation problems, foot ulcers and amputations, blindness, etc.? It is extremely important that, whatever it takes, blood sugar levels be controlled in diabetic patients.

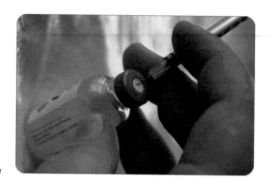

For the most part, insulin is injected into the body using either a needle and syringe or a pen. With a needle and syringe, the insulin comes in vials and is drawn up into the syringe and injected subcutaneously. A pen is actually a hidden needle with the appropriate amount of medication inside. It has a needle inside and is injected subcutaneously as well. An insulin pump delivers insulin 24 hours a day through a catheter under the skin. Traditionally, insulin pumps have been used by people with type 1 diabetes. However, in recent years individuals with type 2 diabetes have been using insulin pumps as well.

There are a number of different types of insulin. They can be synthetic—man-made in a laboratory but otherwise identical to human insulin—or they can come from animals. They can act quickly or take a long time to go into effect. And a number of different drug companies make a variety of brand name insulins.

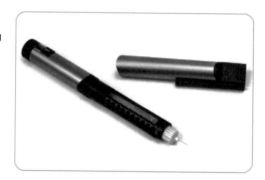

Rapid-acting insulin: takes effect in about five minutes, peaks at an hour, lasts for 2–4 hours.

Regular or short-acting insulin: takes effect within 30 minutes, peaks in 2–3 hours, and lasts for 3–6 hours.

Intermediate-acting insulin: takes effect 2–4 hours after injection, peaks at 4–12 hours, lasts for 12–18 hours.

Long-acting insulin: takes effect 6–10 hours after injection, lasts 20–24 hours.

There are more than 20 different kinds of insulin. Following are a few of the more common ones that you will see in medical reports. They all contain the same generic name *insulin,* such as NPH human insulin or insulin aspart.

- **Humulin** [N, R, 70/30]
- **NovoLog** FlexPen
- **Humalog** [75/25]
- **Lente** and **Ultralente**
- **Lantus & Apidra**

When insulin is dictated as medication in a report, the physician will often dictate a letter or some numbers following the name of the insulin. Notice the contents of the brackets above. These are part of the name of the insulin that is being prescribed and should be edited as dictated. For example:

- Humulin N
- Humulin 70/30
- Humalog 75/25

If the physician dictates a brand name and you are unfamiliar with what follows it or cannot hear it clearly, go to the brand website. The website will generally list all of the different types of that medication that are available. The correct way to edit a brand name medication is always the way that the company selling it has it on their site or on the box, bottle, or vial itself.

Multiple Choice.

Choose the best answer.

1. Insulin pumps are used by people with (○ type 1 diabetes, ○ type 2 diabetes, ○ type 1 and type 2 diabetes) .

2. Insulin (○ lowers, ○ raises) blood sugar levels.

3. (○ Short-acting, ○ Rapid-acting) insulin takes effect fastest.

4. Intermediate-acting insulin lasts (○ 12-18, ○ 20-24) hours after injection.

5. Insulin is usually administered (○ orally, ○ subcutaneously) .

Matching.

Match the second half of the insulin name to the correct first half. Answers may be used more than once or not at all.

1. ____ FlexPen   A. Humulin

2. ____ 70/30   B. Humalog

3. ____ 75/25   C. Novolog

4. ____ N

5. ____ R

THYROID HORMONES

Another set of hormones important to normal body function is released by the thyroid gland. These hormones tell every cell in the body how fast or slow they should be "going." Obviously, these hormones play a significant role in metabolism, which, you remember, means all the chemical processes in the body. The **thyroid hormones** tell all the chemical processes the rate at which they should be functioning.

When the thyroid is not functioning at all or not functioning enough, it leads to feelings of fatigue, cold, dry skin, hair loss, constipation, brittle fingernails, a slowed heart rate, leg cramps, sore muscles, depression, weight gain, and the list goes on. This condition is called **hypothyroidism** (hypo- meaning under or slow).

By the same token, when the rate is revved up, it's not good for the body either. Hyperthyroidism is what happens when the thyroid is overactive (hyper- meaning excessive) and producing too much hormone, i.e., the rate is too high. This can lead to rapid heartbeat, tremors, weakness, hot flashes, weight loss, mood swings, frequent bowel movements. Basically, everything on the list for hypothyroidism but in reverse.

To treat low thyroid, synthetic forms of thyroid hormones are administered in prescription form. The most common of these is **levothyroxine**. It is sold under the brand names **Synthroid** and **Levoxyl**. Another brand name drug Cytomel uses a different generic form of the thyroid hormone, which is more potent than levothyroxine.

Administering more of the thyroid hormone is not what you need when your body is already making too much. Hyperthyroidism tends to be treated with beta blockers or drugs like **propylthiouracil**, which decreases the amount of hormone produced by the thyroid gland.

True/False.
Mark the following true or false.

1. Hyperthyroidism and hypothyroidism can be treated by the same drugs.

   ○ true

   ○ false

2. Some symptoms of hyperthyroidism are rapid heartbeat, weakness, and hot flashes.

   ○ true

   ○ false

3. Hypothyroidism is treated with synthetic forms of thyroid hormones.

   ○ true

   ○ false

4. Levoxyl is used to treat hyperthyroidism.

   ○ true

   ○ false

5. Cytomel is a brand name for levothyroxine.

   ○ true

   ○ false

Spelling.
Determine if the following words are spelled correctly. If the spelling is correct, leave the word as it has already been entered. If the spelling is incorrect, retype the word with the correct spelling. Pay special attention to capitalization.

1. levothyroxane _____

2. propylthioracil _____

3. levoxyl _____

4. Cytomel _____

5. Synthoyd _____

SEX HORMONES

Perhaps the most famous of all hormones are those related to sexuality and reproduction in the human body. Both males and females produce sex hormones, although they are very different and they do very different things in the body. The adrenal glands produce a small amount, but most come from the sex organs themselves (the ovaries and the testes).

A lot of what the sex hormones do you learned about in elementary school sex education: lower the voice, grow hair in new places, induce menstruation, develop breasts, etc. All of this is, of course, in preparation for adulthood and the ultimate goal of propagating the species. It follows, therefore, that most sex hormones used as medication are used in regards to reproduction: infertility, fertility, pregnancy, and lactation.

Because women's bodies actually do all the work when it comes to reproduction, most of the sex hormone medications are comprised of women's hormones and are prescribed to women. However, men also produce sex hormones—most notably **testosterone**—and its lack or overabundance can cause problems requiring medication. Women also produce testosterone, although typically men produce 8–10 times the amount that women do. Testosterone is responsible for libido and protection against osteoporosis. It also reduces the elimination of protein from the body, causing an increase in muscle size.

In women, the primary sex hormones are **estrogen** and **progesterone**. Along with a few others, these hormones tell the female body when to ovulate, build up the appropriate uterine lining, and generally prepare the body for pregnancy. Birth control pills combine some form of either estrogen and progesterone or only progesterone and prevent a woman's body from getting pregnant.

In fact, since the FDA approved "the pill" in 1960, it is the most popular and one of the most effective forms of birth control. More than 18 million U.S. women rely on birth control pills for contraception, and they have more than 40 different ones to choose from, including **Ortho-Novum**, **Ortho Tri-Cyclen**, and recently FDA-approved **Lybrel**, which not only prevents pregnancy, but eliminates menstruation as well. Additionally, the hormones traditionally used in the pill can be put in IUDs or injected IM as well, such as with **Depo-Provera**.

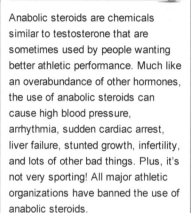

Highlights

Anabolic steroids are chemicals similar to testosterone that are sometimes used by people wanting better athletic performance. Much like an overabundance of other hormones, the use of anabolic steroids can cause high blood pressure, arrhythmia, sudden cardiac arrest, liver failure, stunted growth, infertility, and lots of other bad things. Plus, it's not very sporting! All major athletic organizations have banned the use of anabolic steroids.

In addition to being used as a contraceptive, some forms of estrogen and progesterone are used to treat endometriosis, uterine bleeding, breast cancer, and a number of symptoms of menopause.

Multiple Choice.
Choose the correct spelling of the term.

1. A brand name of a birth control drug.
   - ○ Depo-Povera
   - Depro-Povera
   - Depro-Provera
   - Depo-Provera

2. A primary sex hormone in women.
   - estrogen
   - estragen
   - estragin
   - estrogin

3. A brand name of a birth control drug.
   - Orthronovum
   - Orthro-Novum
   - Ortho-Novum
   - Ortho-Novrum

4. A primary sex hormone in men.
   - testosterone
   - testosteron
   - testostarone
   - testostaron

5. A brand name of a birth control drug.
   - Ortho Tri-Cyclic
   - Ortho Tri-Cyclin
   - Ortho Tri-Cyclen
   - Ortho Tri-Cyclec

6. A brand name of a recently approved birth control drug that prevents pregnancy and eliminates menstruation.
   - Lybrel
   - Librel
   - Libryl
   - Lybril

7. A primary sex hormone in women.
   - progestarone
   - progestrone
   - progesterone
   - progestorone

PREGNANCY AND HORMONES

When the sex hormones are ultimately successful in achieving their purpose, a woman becomes pregnant and more hormones become important. Right away after conception, the body starts to produce increasing amounts of both progesterone and estrogen. In addition, the body starts to make the hormone **HCG (human chorionic gonadotropin)**. This one is credited with all the symptoms of early pregnancy.

The hormone **oxytocin** is released during labor and immediately after a baby is born. It both distends the cervix and induces lactation. Because of its effectiveness, a synthetic form sold under the trade name **Pitocin** is frequently used to both induce and augment labor.

Another drug used to induce labor is **Cytotec**, which has the remarkable ability to ripen the cervix. The pill itself can actually be placed directly in the vagina. Because it is so powerful, it can cause uterine rupture and so is usually broken into pieces. And it is a pretty small pill to begin with!

Multiple Choice.
Choose the best answer.

1. During pregnancy, the body produces (○ more, ○ less) estrogen and progesterone.

2. (○ Progesterone, ○ Human chorionic gonadotropin) is responsible for most or all of the early symptoms of pregnancy.

3. (○ Oxytocin, ○ Pitocin) is a hormone released by the mother during labor.

4. Oxytocin (○ prevents, ○ induces) lactation.

5. (○ Estragen, ○ Estrogen) is produced by the ovaries.

6. (○ Human chorionic gonadotropin, ○ Pitocin) is frequently used to induce labor.

7. The brand name for oxytocin is (○ Pitocin, ○ Pictocin).

8. (○ Cytotec, ○ Cytotek) can be used to induce labor.

9. Oxytocin is released during (○ labor, ○ pregnancy).

INFERTILITY AND HORMONES

The hormones discussed in the preceding pages are what come into play when everything works as it should, and, for the most part, patients are not ever aware of the hormones' actions. However, when things don't work properly, patients are acutely aware of all the sex hormones and exactly how they work. This is because they are catapulted into the world of infertility.

Usually, the first drug used in the treatment of infertility is the generic **clomiphene**, sold under the brand name **Clomid**. It is used to induce ovulation or fix irregular ovulation and helps increase egg production. It works by tricking the pituitary gland into producing more of the follicle-stimulating hormones. It is very effective with female-factor infertility, specifically when the cause involves ovulation, and it usually works quickly. If it doesn't work in the first six months, chances are good that it won't work at all and more extreme measures will need to be taken.

There have been amazing strides in treatments for infertility in the last 30 years. The first "test tube baby" was born on July 25, 1978. Her name is Louise Brown. It's actually been long enough now that she has a baby of her own. She was conceived as a result of a process that is fairly commonplace today called IVF (in vitro fertilization). More than one million children have been conceived using this procedure. A number of hormone-based drugs have been developed to facilitate conception outside the womb and subsequent successful transfer to the uterus.

Remember how estrogen and progesterone are hormones that play an important role in reproduction? There is actually more than one estrogen; and the most common estrogen is called **estradiol**. It is measured during and is an important part of infertility diagnosis and treatment. There are a few other hormones that fall into this category: **LH (luteinizing hormone)** and **FSH (follicle-stimulating hormone)**. All of these hormones are used in IVF and can be purchased under a variety of different brand names, including:

- Follistim
- Repronex
- Pergonal

When an IVF is performed, the first thing that the doctors do is try to gain control of the hormones released naturally. This is so that they can more totally manipulate them. This is accomplished using a drug called **Lupron**. It is used to decrease the body's production of hormone. At that point, all of the drugs necessary for conception are reintroduced synthetically. This includes progesterone, estradiol, LH, and FSH. The object is to "grow" as many healthy eggs as possible at one time.

Because the entire conception process is being manipulated, it is also necessary to synthetically introduce the hormone HCG to release the eggs from the stalks. The most common brand name for this injectable drug is **Pregnyl**.

Multiple Choice.
Choose the best answer.

1. The first drug used in the treatment of infertility is usually (○ clomiphene, ○ Pregnyl).

2. (○ Estrodiol, ○ Estradiol) is the most common estrogen.

3. (○ Clomid, ○ Lupron) is the brand name for clomiphene.

4. Lupron is used to (○ increase, ○ decrease) the body's production of hormone.

5. LH and FSH are examples of (○ insulin, ○ sex hormones).

REVIEW: ENDOCRINE DRUGS

Matching.
Match the correct medications to their trade name.

1. ____ insulin
2. ____ "the pill"
3. ____ metformin
4. ____ furosemide
5. ____ HCG
6. ____ levothyroxine
7. ____ spironolactone
8. ____ oxytocin
9. ____ clomiphene
10. ____ glyburide

A. Glucophage
B. Micronase
C. Synthroid
D. Aldactone
E. Lasix
F. Humulin
G. Pregnyl
H. Pitocin
I. Ortho Tri-Cyclen
J. Clomid

True/False.
Mark the following true or false.

1. Hypothyroidism is when the thyroid does not function at all or enough.

   ○ true

   ○ false

2. Insulin is secreted by the pancreas.

   ○ true

   ○ false

3. Hormones use nerve impulses to transmit messages throughout the body.

   ○ true

   ○ false

4. Estradiol is the most common form of estrogen.

   ○ true

   ○ false

5. Only men produce testosterone.

   ○ true

   ○ false

IMMUNE DRUGS

Immune drugs are what are commonly used to treat a variety of infections, from bacterial to viral. They are very common—you've likely heard of a great many of them. There are several different categories of immune drugs, and we will cover the following:

- Anti-infectives
- Penicillins
- Cephalosporins
- Erythromycins and Tetracyclines
- Antivirals and Antifungals
- Cytotoxics

ANTI-INFECTIVES

Anti-infective drugs are those capable of either slowing the spread of or killing infectious agents. These would include antibiotics, antifungals, antiparasitics, and antiviral drugs.

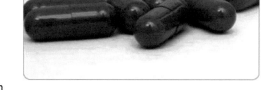

You are probably familiar with the term **antibiotics**. It refers to those drugs that kill or injure bacteria, which are one-celled microorganisms. Bacteria are present all throughout the human body and are mostly harmless. However, some of them cause infectious disease and cause pain, illness, and even death. Drugs that kill bacteria are also sometimes called antibacterials (for obvious reasons). They are one of the most frequently prescribed medications in modern medicine.

The most famous antibiotic is **penicillin**, which was accidentally discovered in molds and first used to treat infection in the 1940s. Its introduction made a major impact upon our society. Prior to the appearance of antibiotics, many diseases and illnesses had no treatment and could be fatal, including simple wound infections and pneumonia. Treatment used to consist of cutting off the offending limb. (Think soldiers on the battlefield prior to World War II, more of whom died from infection than actually in battle.)

Death via an infection (or blood poison) was commonplace 100 years ago. In fact, in the United States, fatal bacterial infections are 1/20 what they were prior to the discovery of antibiotics. In addition, most surgical procedures performed today would simply not be possible without antibiotics to fight potential infection from opening up the body.

Some antibiotics are effective against only one or a few types of bacteria. Others, called **broad-spectrum** antibiotics, are effective against many different kinds of bacteria. The truth is that there are lots and lots of antibiotics effective against a huge variety of different bacteria. It will not be necessary for you to know and understand which types of antibiotics should be used to treat specific diseases, illnesses, or infections. You should only worry about becoming familiar with these terms; you will see them over and over again in medical reports.

PENICILLINS

Let's start with penicillin, since we've already talked a little about it. It is still commonly prescribed to treat a variety of infections. It is considered a class of antibiotics; it can be combined with other compounds, and there are different kinds of penicillin. A few of the most common of these are:

- amoxicillin
- ampicillin
- dicloxacillin
- nafcillin
- piperacillin

Notice that penicillins end in "cillin" and in the generic form, these are all spelled the same.

CEPHALOSPORINS

These are a group of broad-spectrum antibiotics that are similar to penicillin but are used on strains of bacteria that have become resistant to penicillin. There are many individual antibiotics which comprise this group.

Generic examples of cephalosporins include:

- cefuroxime
- ceftazidime
- cephalexin
- ceftriaxone

Some brand name cephalosporins include:

- Ceclor
- Keflex
- Rocephin

Spelling.
Determine if the following words are spelled correctly. If the spelling is correct, leave the word as it has already been entered. If the spelling is incorrect, retype the word with the correct spelling. Pay special attention to capitalization.

1. cefuroxime _____

2. Kephlex _____

3. ceftrixone _____

4. ceftazidine _____

5. Rocefin _____

MACROLIDES AND TETRACYCLINE

Macrolides are antibiotics commonly prescribed to patients with an allergy to penicillins. They are effective against a wide variety of microorganisms but are primarily prescribed to treat pulmonary infections. These drug types actually reduce production of proteins, which bacteria need to survive, and this slows the growth of or even kills the bacteria. The most common macrolides are **Zithromax (azithromycin)**, **Biaxin (clarithromycin)**, and **erythromycin**.

Clindamycin, an antibiotic that works similar to macrolides, is in a class of its own (lincosamides).

Tetracyclines refer to a group of antibiotics, which includes **doxycycline** (sold commonly under the brand name **Vibramycin**), that are a broad-spectrum antibiotic. Unfortunately, their effectiveness has diminished somewhat in recent years due to bacterial resistance, although it remains useful against some bacteria.

This is not to be confused with a specific antibiotic called **tetracycline**, which is especially useful in the treatment of acne. It is sold under a variety of brand names. The specific drug "tetracycline" is also considered a part of the "tetracyclines" group.

Multiple Choice.
Choose the best answer.

1. (○ Macrolides, ○ Tetracyclines) are typically used when a patient has an allergy to penicillin.
2. The generic name for Vibramycin is (○ doxycycline, ○ tetracycline).
3. Drugs that are related to erythromycin act by reducing the production of (○ sugars, ○ proteins) in bacteria.
4. (○ Tetracycline, ○ Zithromax) is useful in the treatment of acne.
5. The effectiveness of tetracyclines has (○ increased, ○ decreased) over the years.

Matching.
Match the drug to its antibiotic group.

1. ____ azithromycin
2. ____ doxycycline
3. ____ tetracycline
4. ____ Zithromax
5. ____ Vibramycin
6. ____ erythromycin

A. macrolides
B. tetracyclines

QUINOLONES AND OTHER ANTIBIOTICS

Quinolones are another class of broad-spectrum antibiotics that work on bacteria by making it difficult or impossible to repair their DNA. They are among the drugs of choice for ophthalmic infections, upper respiratory infections, urinary tract infections, and some sexually transmitted diseases.

A common quinolone is **Cipro (ciprofloxacin)**, an antibiotic that works on bacteria by making it difficult or impossible to repair their DNA. It is also the drug of choice in the treatment of anthrax. Two other common quinolones include **Levaquin (levofloxacin)** and **Avelox (moxifloxacin)**.

There are many other antibiotics frequently used in the treatment of infection and other microorganism invasion. A few of these include the following:

metronidazole, brand name Flagyl– This antibiotic is especially effective against infections that do not require oxygen to grow.

gentamicin, brand name Garamycin– Used in the treatment of serious infections, gentamicin cannot be administered enterally. When the drug passes through the liver, it is rendered completely inactive.

vancomycin– Considered a "drug of last resort," vancomycin is a fairly toxic antibiotic used to treat serious infections (usually in the stomach or bowel) that are not responsive to other antibiotics.

Neosporin– Many different antibiotics can be used topically to treat and prevent bacterial infections. Neosporin contains the antibiotics **neomycin, bacitracin, polymyxin B**.

Multiple Choice.
Choose the correctly spelled term.

1. A brand name of an antibiotic that works on bacteria by making it difficult or impossible to repair their DNA.

   ○ Sipro

   ○ Cipro

   ○ Cipiro

   ○ Sipiro

2. A topical antibiotic.

   ○ bacitrasin

   ○ basitracin

   ○ bacitracin

   ○ basitrasin

3. An antibiotic used to treat bacterial infections in the vagina, stomach, skin, joints, and respiratory tract.

   ○ metronidazole

   ○ metranidazole

   ○ metranidazol

   ○ metronidazol

4. A brand name of metronidazole.

   ○ Flagyl

   ○ Flagil

   ○ flagyl

   ○ flagil

5. A fairly toxic antibiotic used to treat serious infections.

   ○ vancamycin

   ○ vancomycin

   ○ vancamicin

   ○ vancomicin

6. A topical antibiotic.

- ○ polymixin B
- ○ polymixine B
- ○ polymyxine B
- ○ polymyxin B

7. A brand name of a topical antibiotic ointment.

- ○ Neosporine
- ○ neosporine
- ○ Neosporine
- ○ Neosporin

8. A brand name of the antibiotic gentamicin.

- ○ Garomycin
- ○ Garamycin
- ○ Garomicin
- ○ Garamicin

ANTIVIRALS AND ANTIFUNGALS

Also included in the category of anti-infective drugs are drugs that treat fungus or viruses. These are called (appropriately) **antivirals** and **antifungals**.

Common fungal infections include athlete's foot, ringworm, jock itch, and thrush (also called *candidiasis*). A fungus called **Malassezia furfur** causes dandruff, and antifungals are often used in dandruff shampoos. Yeasts are also treated with antifungal medication. A few common antifungals are:

Generic Name	Trade Name
nystatin	Mycostatin
miconazole	Monistat
clotrimazole	Lotrimin, Mycelex
fluconazole	Diflucan

Drugs used to treat viruses are called antivirals. Like antibiotics, they are often specifically targeted at certain viruses. These are primarily used to treat herpes viruses (cold sores and genital herpes), hepatitis B and C, the flu, and an entire class of them known as **antiretrovirals** have been developed to treat HIV. Many of these are in development and there will likely be a number of new ones added in the coming years. Several antiviral medications end in "vir," as in **acyclovir**.

True/False.

Mark the following true or false.

1. Antifungals are only administered orally.

   ○ true

   ○ false

2. Micanazole is the correct spelling for the generic form of Monistat.

   ○ true

   ○ false

3. Antifungal medications also can be used to treat yeast infections.

   ○ true

   ○ false

4. Ringworm is caused by a virus.

   ○ true

   ○ false

5. Nystatin is the generic form of Diflucan.

   ○ true

   ○ false

6. Mycelex is the correct spelling for a brand name of clotrimazole.

   ○ true

   ○ false

7. Dandruff is caused by a fungus.

   ○ true

   ○ false

8. Most antivirals end with -ovir.

   ○ true

   ○ false

9. Medications specifically to treat HIV are antiretrovirals.

   ○ true

   ○ false

10. Most antivirals treat a wide range of viral infections.

    ○ true

    ○ false

CYTOTOXICS

Cytotoxics, also called **antineoplastics**, are drugs that kill or damage cells. **Cytotoxics** are used in chemotherapy to treat cancer. They are also used as immunosuppressives —to suppress the immune system such as may be necessary in the treatment of HIV or to prevent rejection of transplanted organs.

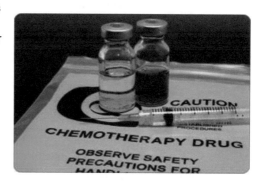

Drugs used in chemotherapy are cytotoxics. What exactly is chemotherapy? Most people know that chemotherapy is used in the treatment of cancer. Normally, cells in the body live through a life cycle and then die; new cells are constantly generated. Cancer is basically when abnormal cells grow and divide to form new cells that are also abnormal, without normal life cycles; in fact, they grow continuously and out of control. Chemotherapy drugs destroy those cells. Unfortunately, they also destroy perfectly healthy cells, especially those that tend to grow rapidly.

It is the destruction of these normal, healthy cells by the chemotherapy drugs that cause the common side effects we hear and see in patients with cancer: nausea and vomiting, hair loss, pain, fatigue. Once the cell-destroying chemotherapy drugs are no longer given, most healthy cells destroyed in the process are able to repair themselves.

A few drugs routinely used as cytotoxics include:

Generic Name	Trade Name
methotrexate	Trexall
ifosfamide	Ifex
doxorubicin	Adriamycin
vincristine	Oncovin

Multiple Choice.
Choose the correct spelling of the term.

1. The brand name of the generic cytotoxic doxorubicin.
   - ○ Adramycin
   - ○ Adriamycin
   - ○ Adramicin
   - ○ Adriamicin

2. The brand name of the generic cytotoxic methotrexate.
   - ○ Trexall
   - ○ Trexal
   - ○ Trixall
   - ○ Trixal

3. A generic cytotoxic.
   - ○ doxorubicin
   - ○ doxirubicin
   - ○ doxorubisin
   - ○ doxirubisin

4. A generic name for the cytotoxic Trexall.
   - ○ methatrexate
   - ○ methitrexate
   - ○ methetrexate
   - ○ methotrexate

5. A generic cytotoxic.
   - ○ ifosfomide
   - ○ iphosfomide
   - ○ ifosphamide
   - ○ ifosfamide

6. A generic name for the cytotoxic Oncovin.
   - ○ vincristine
   - ○ vencristine
   - ○ vincrestine
   - ○ vincristin

7. A brand name of the generic cytotoxic vincristine.
   - ○ Oncovine
   - ○ Oncovin
   - ○ Oncavin
   - ○ Oncavine

REVIEW: IMMUNE DRUGS

Multiple Choice.
Choose the best answer.

1. Some of the most frequently prescribed medications in modern medicine are _____.
   - ○ anti-fungals
   - ○ antibiotics
   - ○ anti-psychotics
   - ○ anti-virals

2. A(n) _____ is an antibiotic that is used on strains of bacteria resistant to penicillin.
   - ○ erythromycin
   - ○ tetracycline
   - ○ cephalosporin
   - ○ Neosporin

3. _____ is a group of antibiotics, as well as a specific antibiotic within that group.
   - ○ tetracycline
   - ○ erythromycin
   - ○ chloramphenicol
   - ○ doxycycline

4. _____ is an antibiotic used to treat anthrax.
   - ○ vancomycin
   - ○ gentamicin
   - ○ metronidazole
   - ○ ciprofloxacin

5. _____ is a toxic antibiotic used as a last resort.
   - ○ vancomycin
   - ○ gentamicin
   - ○ metronidazole
   - ○ ciprofloxacin

6. Anti-viral drugs used to treat HIV are known as _____ .
   - ○ acyclovir
   - ○ nystatin
   - ○ antiretroviral
   - ○ anti-viral plus

7. Cytotoxics are often used in _____.
   - ○ chemotherapy
   - ○ surgery
   - ○ viral infections
   - ○ hormone therapy

8. _____ are drugs that suppress the immune system.

○ chemotherapy

○ immunosuppressives

○ antiretrovirals

○ all of the above

True/False.
Mark the following true or false.

1. Zithromax is a clindamycin.

○ true

○ false

2. Ceclor is a trade name for a cephalosporin.

○ true

○ false

3. Nafcillin is a common kind of penicillin.

○ true

○ false

4. Gentamicin is rendered inactive when it passes through the liver.

○ true

○ false

5. Lotrimin is a trade name of clotrimazole, an antifungal.

○ true

○ false

PAIN MANAGEMENT DRUGS

Pain management drugs do just what they say they do—manage pain. These drugs are essential not only to make a headache go away, but to make certain medical conditions bearable and to make surgery possible. Can you imagine going through an operation without pain medication? Makes you shudder, doesn't it? Of course, there are different categories of pain management drugs, since there are different levels of pain. Here is a list of what we'll be covering:

- Non-narcotic analgesics
- NSAIDs
- Narcotic Analgesics
- Anesthesia
- Corticosteroids

NON-NARCOTIC ANALGESICS

Simply put, analgesics are drugs used to get rid of pain.

There are two main types of analgesics:

1. **Narcotics** or **opioids**. These are derived from the opium poppy, and they go to work on the brain to relieve pain. They also tend to cause drowsiness and a feeling of, for lack of a better word, well-being. Unfortunately, these also tend to be highly addictive.
2. Everything else. This includes aspirin, acetaminophen, ibuprofen, and are often combined with narcotics.

Narcotics tend to be used medically when there is more severe pain. Pain relief for less severe pain has several options. Some of these are nonsteroidal anti-inflammatories (NSAIDs), and they do more than just help with pain. They can also lower fever and reduce swelling. These medicines are probably in one form or another in your own medicine cabinet.

aspirin Originally called acetylsalicylic acid (and this is still accurate), Bayer & Co trademarked the name "Aspirin" in 1899. Its own government denied the application because it was not technically a new product. Bayer's patent was upheld in the United States, however, in 1909, making it 10 times more expensive in the U.S. than in other countries. Germany lost World War I, and the Allies seized Bayer's assets. By 1921 the U.S. established "aspirin" as a genericized trademark. In other countries, there is still a trademark on the name, and they use ASA (a shortened form of acetylsalicylic acid) to refer to the generic.

> **Highlights**
>
> **Genericized trademark**: a brand name that has become colloquial with a particular product or service. Other famous ones: Kleenex, Frisbee, Xerox, Q-tips, Bandaid.

Brand names include: **Bayer, Bufferin, Ecotrin, Excedrin**

acetaminophen Although good at killing pain and lowering fever, acetaminophen is not particularly effective at reducing swelling. Outside of the United States, the most common brand name of this drug is Panadol, and it is marketed under that name in more than 80 countries. It is also the only analgesic that is recommended for use by pregnant women.

Brand names include: **Tylenol, Anacin-3**

ibuprofen Ibuprofen is a nonsteroidal anti-inflammatory developed in the 1960s. While it is an effective pain reliever and fever reducer, unlike acetaminophen it is also highly useful for reducing redness and swelling. It can be classified as either an analgesic or an NSAID, as it is commonly used both to relieve pain and reduce swelling.

Brand names include: **Advil, Motrin, Nuprin, PediaCare**

naproxen This is also a nonsteroidal anti-inflammatory used to alleviate pain, fever, and swelling. It is commonly used for conditions such as arthritis. In most of the world it is a prescription-only pain medication, although in the United States it began to be marketed OTC under the brand name **Aleve**.

Brand names include: **Naprosyn, Anaprox**

True/False.
Mark the following true or false.

1. Narcotics are the most common analgesics, and are sold in most stores.

    ○ true

    ○ false

2. NSAID is an abbreviation for nonsteroidal anti-inflammatory drug.

    ○ true

    ○ false

3. "Bayer" is a genericized trademark referring to acetylsalicylic acid.

    ○ true

    ○ false

4. Ibuprofen and naproxen are generally recommended for pregnant women to take.

    ○ true

    ○ false

5. Acetaminophen is the generic name for Tylenol.

    ○ true

    ○ false

Spelling.
Determine if the following words are spelled correctly. If the spelling is correct, leave the word as it has already been entered. If the spelling is incorrect, retype the word with the correct spelling. Pay special attention to capitalization.

1. Naprosyn _____

2. Bayar _____

3. ibuprophen _____

4. nonsteroidial _____

5. Asprin _____

NSAIDS

NSAID is an acronym for "nonsteroidal anti-inflammatory drugs." When dictated, and it is frequently dictated, it sounds like "en-seds." So, what do these drugs do in the body? They fight inflammation. Inflammation is the body's natural response to injury. Basically, it is the body's way of protecting itself and beginning to heal the wound, injury, or foreign body. Inflammation associated with conditions such as arthritis fits this definition perfectly; for example, when cartilage deteriorates and causes bones to rub together, there is inflammation. For a patient, that means swelling, pain, heat or fever, redness, and sometimes itching. You can certainly see the need for an entire class of drugs to relieve these symptoms. NSAIDs help to alleviate all of these symptoms.

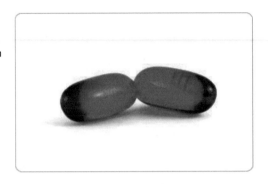

Of course, the name of this drug category is not only anti-inflammatories, but *nonsteroidal* anti-inflammatories. Are there *steroidal* anti-inflammatories, then? Absolutely! And they are regularly used to treat inflammation. Obviously, containing steroids would preclude a drug from being categorized as an NSAID.

Ibuprofen and **naproxen** are commonly prescribed NSAIDs. Of course, you learned about them under analgesics because they are just as frequently used to address the symptom of pain as to address symptoms of inflammation and redness. A number of common drugs, including Advil, Motrin, Nuprin, Anaprox, and Naprosyn, contain ibuprofen and naproxen and are used to treat inflammation.

In addition, the following are commonly prescribed to treat both inflammation and pain:

Generic Name	Trade Name
indomethacin	Indocin
piroxicam	Feldene
tolmetin	Tolectin
nabumetone	Relafen
diclofenac sodium	Voltaren

Matching.
Match the generic name to the trade name.

1. ____ diclofenac sodium
2. ____ indomethacin
3. ____ nabumetone
4. ____ piroxicam
5. ____ tolmetin

A. Feldene
B. Indocin
C. Relafen
D. Tolectin
E. Voltaren

Spelling.
Determine if the following words are spelled correctly. If the spelling is correct, leave the word as it has already been entered. If the spelling is incorrect, retype the word with the correct spelling. Pay special attention to capitalization.

1. napraxsen _____

2. inflammitory _____

3. Feldene _____

4. Nupran _____

5. nalbumatone _____

NARCOTIC ANALGESICS

You are probably already familiar with several narcotics. Because of their addictive nature, they tend to be talked about in the news. Narcotics are prescribed for moderate to severe pain. They are also used during surgery. The following list contains a few of the generic opioids.

> hydrocodone
> codeine
> oxycodone
> morphine
> methadone
>
> propoxyphene
> tramadol
> meperidine
> fentanyl

Most narcotic medications are not purely opioid; they're mixtures of opioids and other ingredients, designed to effectively alleviate pain. Most brand-name narcotic medications fall into this category. Narcotic medications are dispensed as tablets or intravenously, as liquid solutions.

Following is a list of brand name narcotic medications. Although it lists what type of generic medication they are and what other ingredients they contain, you will only be doing exercises on the name of the medication itself and how to spell it.

Terminology.
Enter each term in the space provided. Read the definition and description for each term.

1. Percocet _____

oxycodone and acetaminophen

2. Tylox _____

oxycodone and acetaminophen

3. OxyContin _____

oxycodone

4. Percodan _____

aspirin and oxycodone

5. Vicodin _____

hydrocodone and acetaminophen

6. Lorcet _____

hydrocodone and acetaminophen

7. Darvon _____

propoxyphene

8. Ultram _____

tramadol

9. Demerol _____

meperidine

10. MS-Contin _____

morphine

Multiple Choice.
Choose the correctly spelled term.

1. A generic drug paired with acetaminophen to make Percocet.

   ○ oxicodone

   ○ oxycodone

   ○ oxacodon

   ○ oxycodon

2. A generic name for Ultram.

   ○ tramadal

   ○ trammadol

   ○ trammadal

   ○ tramadol

3. A generic narcotic used to treat pain.

   ○ hydrocodon

   ○ hydrocodone

   ○ hydracodone

   ○ hydracodon

4. A common name of the pain relief narcotic Duragesic.

   ○ fentanyl

   ○ fentanil

   ○ fantenyl

   ○ fantinyl

5. A generic narcotic used to treat pain.

   ○ codene

   ○ codiene

   ○ codeine

   ○ codien

6. The generic name of the brand name narcotic MS Contin.

   ○ morphine

   ○ morphyne

   ○ morphene

   ○ morphin

7. A generic narcotic used to treat pain.

   ○ methadon

   ○ methidone

   ○ methedone

   ○ methadone

8. A generic name of the brand name narcotic Darvon.

   ○ propoxaphene

   ○ prophoxapene

   ○ propoxyphene

   ○ proproxyphene

9. A generic name of the brand name narcotic Demerol.

   ○ meperidine

   ○ mepiridine

   ○ meparidine

   ○ meperedine

ANESTHESIA

Anesthesia is what allows stitches to be put in, bones to be set, and a knife to cut into your skin without pain. The term refers to a loss of pain and sensation through the use of drugs. **Anesthetics** are the drugs that are used to prevent you from feeling. You are probably already familiar with the term "anesthesia" and have had some experience with it. At some point or another, you may have watched in wonder as a needle repeatedly passed through the jagged edges of a formerly painful wound but you felt nothing. Without anesthesia, many medical procedures would simply not be possible or would be excruciatingly painful.

There are three main types of anesthesia.

1. Local anesthesia
2. Regional anesthesia
3. General anesthesia

Local anesthesia numbs only one specific area of the body. Just like in drug effects, it is used when only a small affected area requires treatment. A laceration requiring stitches would necessitate the use of a local anesthetic. A tooth extraction would use local anesthetic. Skin biopsy or removal of a mole is rendered less painful through local anesthesia. This is usually accomplished using a needle injection, ointment, or spray.

Regional anesthesia is used to numb a larger area, although not the entire body, and is accomplished by injecting the anesthetic near a cluster of nerves. This includes an epidural, which numbs the torso during labor and delivery, an interscalene block for spinal surgery, or a femoral nerve block for leg surgery. Many of the same drugs are used to accomplish both local and regional anesthesia.

Some of these include:

Generic Name	Trade Name
procaine	Novocain
lidocaine	Xylocaine
bupivacaine	Marcaine or Sensorcaine
benzocaine	Orajel

General anesthesia is the ultimate in pain relief. That's because it's more or less oblivion. You not only feel no pain but also no sensation whatsoever, and you remember nothing to boot. In fact, patients often are unable to breathe on their own under general anesthesia and require intubation for assistance in respiration. General anesthesia can be administered via IV or inhalation, or some combination of the two. It has three basic components: an analgesic for relief of pain; a paralytic for loss of sensation, muscle tone, and reflex movement; and an amnesic, to prevent the formation of any memory of the event. It is not uncommon for one drug to accomplish more than one of these objectives. Many of the drugs you learned about in Analgesics could be used in combination with anesthetics to achieve the overall result.

General anesthesia is used primarily during surgery, although it can also be used after serious injury or trauma so the patient does not have to feel or remember their pain and discomfort. Surgery would simply not be possible without all of the components of general anesthesia. There are several different drugs and combinations of drugs used to achieve general anesthesia. A few of these include:

Inhalational:

- nitrous oxide
- halothane
- desflurane

Intravenous:

Generic Name	Trade Name
methohexital	Brevital
midazolam	Versed
propofol	Diprivan

Some of these are straight anesthetics, and others, like midazolam, are an antianxiety, amnesic, hypnotic, muscle relaxant, and sedative all rolled into one.

Multiple Choice.
Choose the correctly spelled term.

1. A generic form of the drug Novocain.

   ○ procane

   ○ procain

   ○ procan

   ○ procaine

2. An inhalational anesthesia.

   ○ nitrous oxite

   ○ nitrus oxite

   ○ nitrous oxide

   ○ nitrous oxiod

3. A loss of pain and sensation through the use of drugs.

   ○ anesthesia

   ○ anasthesia

   ○ anesthasia

   ○ anisthesia

4. An intravenous anesthesia.

   ○ methahexital

   ○ methohexital

   ○ methahexitol

   ○ methohexitol

5. A generic name for the regional anesthesia Xylocaine.

   ○ lidacaine

   ○ lidacain

   ○ lidocaine

   ○ lidocain

6. A brand name of the local anesthesia benzocaine.

   ○ Orajel

   ○ Orojel

   ○ Oragel

   ○ Orogel

7. A brand name of the generic anesthesia lidocaine.

   ○ Xylocain

   ○ Xylacain

   ○ Xylocaine

   ○ Xylacaine

8. A generic name of an intravenous anesthesia.

   ○ midazolam

   ○ medazolam

   ○ midazalam

   ○ medazalam

9. A brand name of the intravenous anesthesia propofol.

   ○ Diprovan

   ○ Dipravan

   ○ Dipravam

   ○ Diprivan

10. A brand name of the intravenous anesthesia midazolam.

   ○ Versed

   ○ Verssed

   ○ Varsed

   ○ Varssed

CORTICOSTEROIDS

Now that you know about nonsteroidal anti-inflammatory medications, what about the steroidal ones? Are these those "steroids" that athletes are forever getting in trouble for using to "juice up"? Nope. Those are called anabolic steroids. The steroids that your doctor may prescribe to fight inflammation (and treat a number of other conditions) are called **corticosteroids**.

They are so called because they are similar to cortisol, a hormone naturally produced in the adrenal glands. In fact, they are so similar that your body can't tell the difference between a corticosteroid that you take externally and the cortisol that your body naturally produces. It is sometimes called the stress hormone because your body produces cortisol when it's under stress—really any kind of stress, including surgery, emotional strain, infection, trauma. When the stressful situation ends, the adrenals stop producing as much cortisol.

The nice thing about corticosteroids is that not only are they good at fighting inflammation, they are effective at treating a number of medical conditions, including preventing organ rejection in transplant recipients. When they were first introduced in the 1950s, they were considered a miracle drug. They virtually eliminated any symptoms of arthritis, and many people thought that they were a permanent cure for the condition. The problem is that prolonged use of corticosteroids causes the body to quit making cortisol on its own. This condition is called "adrenal suppression." It, along with other side effects, causes these drugs to be prescribed in tapering doses.

> **Highlights**
>
> Corticosteroids are used to treat:
>
> - arthritis (juvenile, rheumatoid)
> - lupus
> - ankylosing spondylitis
> - inflammatory bowel disease
> - Addison's disease
> - scleroderma
> - asthma
> - Crohn's disease

All of the common generic corticosteroid drugs end in either -sone or -olone, making it another one of those really easy-to-remember drug categories. It makes it easy to look up difficult-to-understand terms a physician may dictate—if it sounds like it ends in either of the above ways, look up corticosteroids and see if you can identify the drug that was dictated that way.

The most commonly prescribed corticosteroid is **prednisone**. However, there are a number of others, all of which you may see when editing medical reports. In alphabetic order:

Generic Name	Trade Name
betamethasone	Luxiq
beclomethasone	Qvar
cortisone	Cortone Acetate
dexamethasone	Decadron
fluocinolone	Retisert
hydrocortisone	Nutracort
methylprednisolone	Medrol
triamcinolone	Kenalog

Multiple Choice.
Choose the best answer.

1. Corticosteroids are used to treat (◯ arthritis, ◯ skin infections).

2. Corticosteroids can be used (◯ indefinitely, ◯ for a limited time).

3. Generic corticosteroids usually end in (◯ -olone, ◯ -alone) or -sone.

4. The generic form of Nutracort is (◯ hydrocortisone, ◯ prednisone).

5. Corticosteroids are very similar to the (◯ adrenaline, ◯ cortisol) that the body produces when stressed.

Matching.

Match the generic drug to its brand name.

1. ____ betamethasone

2. ____ cortisone

3. ____ dexamethasone

4. ____ methylprednisolone

5. ____ triamcinolone

A. Cortone Acetate

B. Decadron

C. Kenalog

D. Luxiq

E. Medrol

REVIEW: PAIN MANAGEMENT DRUGS

Fill In The Blank.
Enter the correct word in the blank provided.

1. Narcotics are derived from the _____ poppy.

2. NSAIDs stand for _____ anti-inflammatories.

3. NSAIDs are used often because _____ is the body's natural response to injury.

4. Most _____ are mixtures of opioids and other ingredients.

5. _____ anesthesia numbs one specific area of the body.

6. A general anesthetic includes an analgesic, a paralytic, and an _____

7. Steroids used to treat inflammation are called _____

8. The most commonly prescribed corticosteroid is _____

Matching.
Match the correct generic name to the brand name.

1. ____ naproxen

2. ____ acetaminophen

3. ____ cortisone

4. ____ aspirin

5. ____ tolmetin

6. ____ nabumetone

7. ____ tramadol

8. ____ morphine

9. ____ lidocaine

10. ____ midazolam

A. Aleve

B. Tolectin

C. MS-Contin

D. Xylocaine

E. Ultram

F. Excedrin

G. Tylenol

H. Relafen

I. Cortone Acetate

J. Versed

PSYCHOLOGICAL DRUGS

Psychological drugs are used in many situations to treat psychological conditions from depression to schizophrenia. These often work on the chemicals in the brain, and fall into these categories:

- Antianxiety
- Antidepressants
- Antipsychotics

ANTIANXIETY

Antianxiety medications are just what they sound like—medications to treat anxiety. In our society, we call these types of drugs by many different names: antianxiety medications, sedatives, tranquilizers, muscle relaxants. The number of terms used to describe basically the same thing should give you an indication of our collective stress level! Of course, I am oversimplifying a bit here. Different types of antianxiety medications work in slightly different ways to solve slightly different problems. For the most part, though, they have a calming effect and work to reduce certain chemicals in the brain.

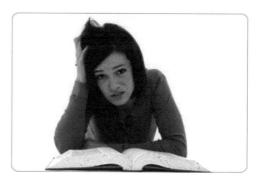

What are some of the most common antianxiety medications?

A class of antianxiety medications that have been common in the treatment of a variety of anxiety disorders for many years is **benzodiazepines**. These are used to treat general anxiety disorders, panic disorder, phobias, insomnia, muscle spasm, alcohol withdrawal, and sometimes seizures. These have a tendency to lead to dependency and abuse. You are familiar with some of these medications.

Generic Name	Trade Name
alprazolam	Xanax
clonazepam	Klonopin
diazepam	Valium
lorazepam	Ativan
triazolam	Halcion

The individual names of generic drugs in this class sound very similar, with a "z" in the middle and an "am" at the end. H2 blockers tend to include "tidi" in the name, and proton pump inhibitors tend to end in "prazole" as well. Recognizing similarities will make it much easier to identify drug categories and help you in your work as an MT. Of course, you may have noticed that all bets are off for the brand names though. This is, in part, what makes drugs a complex area to transcribe.

There is another muscle relaxant which is not related to the benzodiazepines but seems to be as effective in the treatment of anxiety. It has the added benefits of not being prone to dependency and not functioning as a sedative. In its generic form it is known as buspirone and is sold under several different brand names, including **BuSpar**.

Muscle relaxants are also commonly classed as antianxiety medications. A few common brand name muscle relaxants include **Flexeril** and **Norflex**. **Baclofen** (a generic drug) is considered an antispasmodic, to relax spastic or rigid muscles. It is specifically used either for spine muscles, as in spinal cord injury, or with multiple sclerosis and ALS (Lou Gehrig disease).

Multiple Choice.
Choose the correct spelling of the term.

1. Class of drugs that treat general anxiety, insomnia, and panic attacks.

    ○ benzdiazepines

    ○ benzadiazopines

    ○ benzodiazepines

    ○ benzodiazopines

2. ____ is NOT a benzodiazepine.

    ○ alprazolam

    ○ buspirone

    ○ lorazepam

    ○ triazolam

3. A drug used to treat anxiety is ____.

    ○ Zanax

    ○ Xanax

    ○ Zantac

    ○ Xantac

4. A common brand name drug for the benzodiazepine known as diazepam is ____.

    ○ Valium

    ○ valium

    ○ Vallium

    ○ valium

5. A brand name antianxiety medication that is not a benzodiazepine is ____.

    ○ buspar

    ○ BuSpar

    ○ Buspare

    ○ buSpare

6. A generic name antianxiety medication that is not a benzodiazepine is ____.

    ○ buspirone

    ○ buspiron

    ○ Buspirone

    ○ Buspiron

7. A common brand name drug for the benzodiazepine known as clonazepam is ____.

    ○ Clonopin

    ○ Klonopin

    ○ Clonapin

    ○ Klonapin

8. A brand name muscle relaxant.

    ○ Flexoril

    ○ Flexaril

    ○ Flexeril

    ○ Flexiril

9. A brand name benzodiazepine.

    ○ Halceon

    ○ Halcione

    ○ Halsione

    ○ Halcion

10. Drugs to relax muscles, provide relief for panic disorder and anxiety, and treat insomnia are classified as ____.

    ○ antacids

    ○ antianxiety medications

    ○ analgesics

    ○ anesthesia

ANTIDEPRESSANTS

More than 20 million people in the United States suffer from some form of depression. This is considered to be more than just feeling blue or being sad; depression includes a variety of symptoms that last for weeks, months, and even years. These symptoms include feelings of sadness, worthlessness, inability to sleep, disinterest in any activities, weight fluctuation, and in its most extreme form, thoughts of suicide (suicidal ideation). It is not uncommon for women to experience symptoms of depression following the birth of a baby (postpartum depression) or for people to suffer depressive symptoms throughout the long winter months (seasonal affective disorder), and depression can be a component of a number of different, more severe psychiatric disorders, such as obsessive-compulsive disorder (OCD) and bipolar disorder.

Antidepressants work by increasing the production of certain chemicals within the brain, such as serotonin. A multitude of studies have concluded that there is a correlation between the amount of these chemicals present in an individual and his or her mood.

There are so many drugs used to enhance mood and treat depression that I am going to break them up here by grouping them into some common categories:

1. Tricyclic antidepressants
2. SSRIs (selective serotonin reuptake inhibitors)
3. Monoamine oxidase inhibitors
4. Tetracyclic compounds and other types of antidepressants

First, tricyclic antidepressants. These are the oldest type of antidepressants, developed in the 1950s. Although they have largely been replaced in recent years by newer types of drugs, they are still prescribed and are effective against the symptoms of depression, ADHD, migraine headaches, insomnia, and bulimia (to name just a few). They work by inhibiting certain neurotransmitters (namely norepinephrine, dopamine, and serotonin) from re-entering nerve cells, causing levels to increase.

Generic Name	Trade Name
imipramine	Tofranil
desipramine	Norpramin
nortriptyline	Pamelor

Selective serotonin reuptake inhibitors (SSRIs) work essentially the same way but on one specific neurotransmitter, namely serotonin. Although nobody seems to know why, the increase of serotonin levels elevates mood and thus treats a number of depression symptoms.

Generic Name	Trade Name
paroxetine	Paxil
fluoxetine	Prozac
sertraline	Zoloft
venlafaxine	Effexor

Monoamine oxidase inhibitors are extremely powerful antidepressants, with potentially lethal drug and dietary interactions. They have traditionally been used only after tricyclics and SSRIs have been tried without success. However, in 2006, a patch form of an MAOI was approved by the FDA, and since it does not require passage through the gastrointestinal system, it is a much safer form. These types of drugs can be used in the treatment of agoraphobia (fear of different settings, which can cause sufferers to never leave their homes) and social anxiety. They work by preventing the breakdown of the specific neurotransmitter monoamine, increasing its stores. Because it has such potentially harmful side effects, it is not commonly prescribed.

The last category of antidepressants includes tetracyclic compounds and any other antidepressant that does not fit nicely into one of the above categories. It is amazing when reading and learning about the different drugs, some of which have been on the market for 25 years or more, how little is known about how they work or why they work. As a medical transcriptionist, you don't need to understand the details of how antidepressants work; just familiarize yourself with some of these more commonly prescribed drugs and know that they will continue to change as more research is completed.

Generic Name	Trade Name
trazodone	Desyrel
bupropion	Wellbutrin

Antidepressants are also sometimes used for other things, such as antihistamines or to help people quit smoking. In addition, other types of drugs, like benzodiazepines, can be used to treat depression. When editing, you may come across a drug prescribed for depression that you recognize as, say, an antianxiety medicine or a sleeping pill (for example, Xanax). When this happens, you can flag it to the attention of the dictating physician just to make sure it's what he/she intended, or you can do a little research on your own. Look up the drug and see what all of its uses are.

Multiple Choice.
Choose the best answer.

1. Antidepressants are also sometimes used _____.

   ○ as an antihistamine

   ○ to help people quit smoking

   ○ all of the above

   ○ none of the above

2. Antidepressants are usually not prescribed for ____.

   ○ suicidal ideation

   ○ postpartum depression

   ○ obsessive-compulsive disorder

   ○ short-term "blues"

3. Tricyclic antidepressants work by ____ levels of certain neurotransmitters.

   ○ keeping the same

   ○ increasing

   ○ decreasing

   ○ eliminating

4. MAOIs have ____ side effects.

   ○ minimal

   ○ moderate

   ○ potentially lethal

   ○ no

5. SSRI stands for ____.

   ○ selective serotonin reuptake inhibitors

   ○ selective serotonin reduction inhibitors

   ○ selective serotonin reuptake increasers

   ○ standard serotonin reuptake inhibitors

Matching.
Match each drug to its classification. Some answers will be used more than once, or not at all.

1. ____ Prozac   A. tricyclic

2. ____ bupropion   B. SSRI

3. ____ Pamelor   C. MAOI

4. ____ Effexor   D. tetracyclic and others

5. ____ sertraline

ANTIPSYCHOTICS

Antipsychotic medications, also called neuroleptics or major tranquilizers, are typically used for the most severe mental disorders. There are a number of drugs prescribed to patients with varying forms of depression and milder mental conditions. Psychosis, on the other hand, tends to describe mental conditions that are more severe, often involving a loss of contact with reality and significant social impairment; specifically, conditions like bipolar disorder, schizophrenia, delusions, and mania.

The idea behind antipsychotic medication is to calm some areas of the brain while allowing most of it to continue to function normally. The types of symptoms that antipsychotics are trying to mitigate or eliminate include hallucinations, tension, hyperactivity, combativeness, or severe antisocial behavior.

The treatment of patients with these symptoms has changed dramatically since the introduction of antipsychotic medications in the 1950s. How about a short history lesson? In the 1600s, mental illness was attributed to witchcraft or demonic possession, and torture and death were not uncommon "treatments." For the next few hundred years, reason prevailed and those with mental illness were merely locked up, chained up, or left to wander the streets. Fortunately, by the 20th century, society had become enlightened when it came to mental illness. Starting in the 1930s, physicians injected patients suffering from schizophrenia with insulin, putting them into shock and a temporary coma. By 1936, treatment consisted of the frontal lobotomy—more than 20,000 of which were eventually performed in the United States. Electric shock therapy became commonplace for treatment of mental illness in the 1940s. Are you horrified yet?

In 1951 in France, a physician named Henri Laborit used the new drug **chlorpromazine**, brand name **Thorazine**, to reduce anxiety in his patients prior to surgery. It was so calming that he thought it might be effective in patients suffering from mental illness. In fact, it was found to significantly decrease symptoms of agitation without sedation or loss of consciousness. Not only that, but in addition to reducing physical symptoms, patients' thinking became less chaotic. By 1955 it was getting widespread use. As its use increased, the number of mental illness patients living as inpatients in hospitals dramatically decreased.

A number of similar antipsychotic medications have been introduced since Thorazine. In 1957, **haloperidol** was developed as a very potent neuroleptic. By weight it is 50 times more potent than chlorpromazine, and it works against delusions and hallucinations in the treatment of schizophrenia and delirium. Sold under the brand name **Haldol**, it didn't actually receive FDA approval until 1988.

Other antipsychotic medications include:

- clozapine
- olanzapine
- risperidone
- paliperidone
- lithium
- quetiapine

Spelling.
Determine if the following words are spelled correctly. If the spelling is correct, leave the word as it has already been entered. If the spelling is incorrect, retype the word with the correct spelling.

1. haldoperidol _____

2. risporidan _____

3. chlorpromazine _____

4. olansapine _____

5. lithuim _____

6. klozapine _____

7. Thorazeen _____

8. Haldol _____

REVIEW: PSYCHOLOGICAL DRUGS

Multiple Choice.
Choose the best answer.

1. (○ Benzodiazepines, ○ buspirone) are used to treat general anxiety and have a tendency to lead to abuse.

2. SSRI stands for selective (○ sertraline, ○ serotonin) reuptake inhibitors.

3. Antipsychotic medications are also called (○ neurotranquilizers, ○ neuroleptics).

4. Psychological drugs often work on the (○ chemicals, ○ proteins) in the brain.

5. Muscle relaxants are also commonly classed as (○ diabetic, ○ antianxiety) medications.

True/False.
Mark the following true or false.

1. Flexeril is a common muscle relaxant.

   ○ true

   ○ false

2. Antidepressants can sometimes be used as antihistamines.

   ○ true

   ○ false

3. Antipsychotics excite certain areas of the brain while allowing the rest to function normally.

   ○ true

   ○ false

4. The generic name for Prozac is fluoxetine.

   ○ true

   ○ false

5. Chlorpromazine's brand name is Thorazine.

   ○ true

   ○ false

RESPIRATORY DRUGS

If you've ever had a cold, you are probably grateful for this group of drugs! Respiratory drugs are used to treat problems of the respiratory system, helping everything from sniffles to coughs to asthma. Seeing as breathing is a rather essential part of life, these drugs are very important! Here's a list of the categories we will be covering:

- Antihistamines
- Bronchodilators
- Cough suppressants and expectorants
- Decongestants

ANTIHISTAMINES

Antihistamines are drugs that act against histamines. Helpful? Probably not so much. It's a type of medication that you have probably heard quite a bit. What are they? Drugs for allergies? Yes. But what is a histamine? And why do we need to go into battle against them? Believe it or not, histamine is actually a good thing. It helps to regulate physiologic function and works as a neurotransmitter in the brain. In fact, it plays an important role in both sleep and orgasm, neither of which you probably want to live without. In addition, low levels of histamine are correlated with schizophrenia. Less and less something that you want to fight, right?

Well, for some people, normal, innocuous, everyday things like dust or pollen are seen by their bodies as major invaders. So, their "mast cells" send histamine, lots of histamine, to their bodies. Mast cells happen to be particularly numerous at vulnerable places—the nose, mouth, and blood vessels, for example. The histamine creates a chemical response that causes inflammation and smooth muscle constriction. That results in itching, sneezing, runny nose, watery eyes, and asthma. Now you can see the value of diminishing histamines!

Interestingly, because histamines are neurotransmitters as well, antihistamines work in the "vomiting center" of the brain to control nausea and vomiting. So, in addition to controlling allergy symptoms, antihistamines are also effective antiemetics. Scopolamine, meclizine, and dimenhydrinate (the generic form of the drug Dramamine) are antihistamines that are particularly effective at controlling motion sickness. And the drug promethazine, which you learned about in antiemetics, is technically an antihistamine.

Closely related to dimenhydrinate is **diphenhydramine**, the generic form of the drug **Benadryl**. You may have heard of Benadryl. It is a very common over-the-counter allergy medicine used to treat a number of allergic conditions (and colds for that matter).

There are many other over-the-counter antihistamines. These include brompheniramine, which is sold under the brand names **Dimetapp** and **Robitussin** (among others); doxylamine, which is a primary ingredient in **NyQuil**; and loratadine, which is the antihistamine in **Alavert** and **Claritin**.

The generic drug **hydroxyzine** is sold under the names **Vistaril** and **Atarax**. Notice that the sound of the drug is similar to "meclizine," which is classified as an antiemetic. Technically an anxiolytic, hydroxyzine tends to be frequently prescribed as an antihistamine. However, it can also be used to treat motion sickness and as an antianxiety medication because of its effectiveness as a tranquilizer. Remember that histamines are also neurotransmitters, so they have an effect upon the brain.

Other prescription antihistamines include **Allegra**, which is the brand name of fexofenadine, and **Zyrtec**, a common brand name for the generic drug cetirizine.

Notice that in this category, most of the generic forms of the drug have not been bolded. Although you will occasionally see the generic form in medical reports, it is fairly uncommon. Antihistamines are frequently combined with other ingredients in various forms of the brand name drugs. For example, NyQuil contains an antihistamine, but depending on *which form* of NyQuil you take, it can also have acetaminophen to relieve pain and reduce fever, a cough suppressant, and a decongestant. Physicians will usually dictate the name of the specific drug or drugs that were recommended or prescribed and not focus in on one generic antihistamine.

Multiple Choice.
Choose the best answer.

1. Low levels of histamines are associated with _____.

   ○ schizophrenia

   ○ sleep

   ○ immune responses

   ○ orgasm

2. Antihistamines can also function as _____.

   ○ beta blockers

   ○ cytotoxics

   ○ antiemetics

   ○ antidepressants

3. Histamines do not ____.
   - ○ constrict smooth muscles
   - ○ cause inflammation
   - ○ act as a neurotransmitter
   - ○ play a role in digestion

4. The generic form of Benadryl is ____.
   - ○ loratadine
   - ○ diphenhydramine
   - ○ doxylamine
   - ○ meclizine

5. Hydroxyzine is technically classified as a/an ____.
   - ○ antiemetic
   - ○ anxiolytic
   - ○ antianxiety medication
   - ○ neurotransmitter

6. A brand name for fexofenadine is ____.
   - ○ Alegra
   - ○ Alegraa
   - ○ Allegra
   - ○ Allegraa

7. NyQuil usually has an antihistamine and ____.
   - ○ no other drugs
   - ○ acetaminophen or other additional drugs
   - ○ a narcotic
   - ○ an antibiotic

8. The generic form of Zyrtec is ____.
   - ○ hydroxyzine
   - ○ diphenhydramine
   - ○ cetirizine
   - ○ loratadine

9. The generic form of the antihistamine in Robitussin is ____.
   - ○ brompheniramine
   - ○ bromfenaramine
   - ○ bromphenirimine
   - ○ bromfeniramine

10. A brand name for loratadine is ____.
    - ○ Zyrtec
    - ○ Atarax
    - ○ Dimetapp
    - ○ Claritin

BRONCHODILATORS

Bronchodilators do what their name implies they do: dilate the bronchi. They work by relaxing the smooth muscles surrounding the airways. This causes the airways to dilate or widen, making it easier to breathe. They can be used to dilate already constricted airways or to prevent airways from becoming constricted in the first place. Bronchodilators most commonly treat asthma.

Asthma is a chronic lung disease that causes the airways to become swollen and irritated and the muscles around the airways to tighten. This can seriously limit the ability to take in air. An asthma attack can be painful and frightening. Some have compared it to trying to breathe through a coffee stirrer. If you have ever been trapped underwater just a little too long while swimming, you can probably appreciate the panic that accompanies a need to breathe and the inability to get air.

In addition to treating asthma, bronchodilators are used to treat other pulmonary conditions as well, including bronchitis, COPD (chronic obstructive pulmonary disease), emphysema, and pneumonia.

Frequently, bronchodilators are lumped into three main categories: beta-agonists, anticholinergics, and theophyllines.

Beta-agonists can be either "long acting" or "short acting." When they are short acting, they are often called "rescue" medications. This is because they work very quickly (within a few minutes, up to 15–20 minutes) and can be the difference between life and death. A few short-acting beta-agonists include **albuterol**, which is sold under the brand names **Proventil** and **Ventolin**, and **pirbuterol**, sold as **Maxair**.

Long-acting beta-agonists do not work immediately, but their effects last much longer than the short-acting ones. Therefore, they are not used in an emergent situation but are used consistently to open up the airways and keep them open. A common long-acting beta-agonist is **Serevent**.

The second category of bronchodilators is **anticholinergics**. These also do not act right away. They are inhaled regularly to keep the airways open. A common anticholinergic is **ipratropium**, which is sold under the brand name **Atrovent**.

Patients can get a prescription for a home nebulizer, significantly cutting down on emergency room visits in cases of severe asthma.

Sometimes short-acting beta-agonists are combined with anticholinergics to make an even more powerful bronchodilator, as is the case with **Combivent**. It combines albuterol (the beta-agonist) and ipratropium (the anticholinergic).

Bronchodilators are often (although not always) administered to patients via inhalers and nebulizers. These allow small doses of the medicine to be released and breathed in using special equipment. You may remember that nebulizers take a liquid form of a medication and turn it into a vapor, allowing it to be easily ingested. It allows the largest dose to be delivered and thus can provide the fastest relief of symptoms. They are often used in hospitals.

The third and final category of bronchodilators is **theophylline**. Sold under the brand names **Theo-Dur** and **Slo-bid**, it is a long-acting bronchodilator that can be administered via IV or taken in pill form. It is most commonly taken for severe cases of asthma and must be taken daily.

Multiple Choice.
Choose the correct spelling of the term.

1. Drugs that work by relaxing the smooth muscles surrounding the airways.

   ○ bronchadilator

   ○ bronchodilater

   ○ bronchadilator

   ○ bronchodilator

2. A brand name of the short-acting beta-agonist albuterol.

- ○ Proventol
- ○ Proventil
- ○ Provantil
- ○ Provantol

3. A brand name of a long-acting bronchodilator.

- ○ Slow-Bid
- ○ Slo-bid
- ○ Slow-bid
- ○ Slo-Bid

4. Drugs used to open airways.

- ○ betagonist
- ○ betaagonist
- ○ betoagonist
- ○ beta-agonist

5. A brand name of a long-acting beta-agonist.

- ○ Serevent
- ○ Seravent
- ○ Serovent
- ○ Serivent

6. A generic short-acting beta-agonist.

- ○ albuterol
- ○ albuterole
- ○ albeturol
- ○ albeturole

7. A drug combining albuterol and ipratropium.

- ○ Combavent
- ○ Combevent
- ○ Comibavent
- ○ Combivent

8. A type of bronchodilator commonly taken for severe cases of asthma.

- ○ theophalline
- ○ theophylline
- ○ theofylline
- ○ theophyline

9. A generic bronchodilator that is inhaled regularly to keep airways open.

- ○ ipratropium
- ○ ipatropium
- ○ ipratroprium
- ○ ipatroprium

COUGH SUPPRESSANTS AND EXPECTORANTS

Cough suppressant medications control coughs. Another name for cough suppressants is **antitussives**. "Tussive" is just another way to say "cough." You will rarely actually see coughs referred to as tussives, although you will see cough medication referred to as antitussives.

Coughing is actually a reflex—a very good reflex—designed to expel unwanted material (such as mucus) from your breathing passages. In the event that the body has the need of eradicating something from its breathing passages, you don't really want that reflex to be suppressed. In fact, in these instances you want to use an **expectorant**, a drug to stimulate the production of saliva and induce coughing, making it more likely to eliminate whatever is blocking the airways. **Guaifenesin** is used in over-the-counter medications targeted at cold-related symptoms. It works by loosening the mucus or phlegm in the lungs, making them easier to cough up.

On the other hand, when the reflex kicks into gear and there is nothing to expel (resulting in a dry, unproductive cough), it can be very irritating. At that point, you want to suppress the natural coughing reflex. This can be done in a variety of ways. One of the most common medications for cough suppression is **dextromethorphan**, a common ingredient in cold medicines. It works on the brain to suppress the urge to cough. Codeine, which you may remember as a narcotic, also is used as a cough suppressant and works in the same manner.

As opposed to suppressing the cough through drugs that work on the nerves of the brain, coughs can be suppressed by drugs that have a local effect—primarily a local anesthetic on the irritated throat tissues. Examples of antitussives that work locally are **Chloraseptic** and the **menthol** in throat lozenges.

> ### Highlights
>
> Interestingly enough, most over-the-counter cold medicines contain BOTH guaifenesin and dextromethorphan, the goal being to promote and expel the productive cough while simultaneously suppressing the dry, useless cough.

Lots of "medicines" get lumped into this category that are not truly cough suppressants in the sense that they contain no actual medication. Many cough drops, for example, fall into this category. They are primarily sugar, honey, or glycerin. These soothe irritation in the throat basically by keeping it wet, thereby preventing a cough, but they contain no drugs that actually suppress coughing. In fact, you may have noticed that when you have a serious cough, the only time you are not coughing is when the drop is actually in your mouth. The moment it dissolves, you begin coughing again.

True/False.
Mark the following true or false.

1. Coughing is a useless reflex.

   ○ true

   false

2. If someone has a dry cough, they would want an antitussive.

   true

   false

3. There is never a reason to take both a cough suppressant and an expectorant.

   true

   false

4. Codeine works as a cough suppressant.

   true

   false

5. Some antitussives work systemically, while some work locally.

   true

   false

DECONGESTANTS

Decongestants are medications used to relieve nasal congestion or a "stuffy nose." Often a symptom of a cold, congestion occurs when the membranes of the nose become swollen. This is caused by inflamed blood vessels. Anybody who has ever had a stuffy nose is well aware of why medications exist to alleviate this condition!

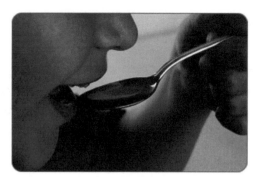

Drugs to treat congestion work by constricting the blood vessels in the nose and sinuses, thereby opening up those nasal passages. Aaah! They are available in a couple of different forms. Oral decongestants are taken by mouth (often as part of a multi-symptom cold medicine) and are slow acting. They do not, however, interfere with either the production of mucus or the movement of cilia (the "hair" that sweeps debris out of air passages). Topical decongestants, which include nasal sprays and nasal drops, provide virtually immediate relief. However, they do tend to slow down the movement of the cilia.

Decongestants are often confused with antihistamines, but they are different. Remember that antihistamines work on the brain to block the production of "histamine" and are an effective weapon against allergies. Decongestants, on the other hand, work to constrict the blood vessels that supply the nose. They are much more limited in scope.

There are really only a few decongestants on the market. First, and one that has been used for a long time, is **pseudoephedrine**, the primary ingredient in **Sudafed**. However, because pseudoephedrine is an ingredient in the illicit drug methamphetamine, it is largely being replaced as an ingredient by the decongestant **phenylephrine**. These are ingredients in a number of cold medicines, which tend to also contain fever reducers, cough suppressants, and other categories of drugs.

Additionally, a number of nasal drips and sprays are decongestants. A couple of these include **Afrin** and **Dristan**.

Multiple Choice.
Choose the best answer.

1. Nasal congestion is the same thing as a (○ stuffy nose, ○ runny nose).
2. Oral decongestants work (○ slowly, ○ quickly).
3. (○ Phenylephrine, ○ Pseudoephedrine) is the main ingredient in Sudafed and methamphetamine.
4. Decongestants work by (○ constricting blood vessels, ○ decreasing mucus production).
5. In addition to orally, decongestants can also be administered (○ auricularly, ○ nasally).

Spelling.
Determine if the following words are spelled correctly. If the spelling is correct, leave the word as it has already been entered. If the spelling is incorrect, retype the word with the correct spelling. Pay special attention to capitalization.

1. pseudoephedrine _____

2. dripstan _____

3. decongestent _____

4. Sudafed _____

5. phenylefrine _____

REVIEW: RESPIRATORY DRUGS

Fill In The Blank.
Enter the correct word in the blank provided.

1. Antihistamines also work well as _____ .

2. Diphenhydramine is the generic form of the drug _____ .

3. _____ are used as "rescue" medications.

4. _____ which is also a narcotic, is used as a cough suppressant.

5. _____ treat congestion by constricting the blood vessels in the nose and sinuses.

Multiple Choice.
Choose the best answer.

1. Histamines work as a (◯ hormone, ◯ neurotransmitter) in the brain.

2. Bronchodilators are often used for (◯ allergies, ◯ asthma).

3. (◯ Anticholinergics, ◯ Theophylline) bronchodilators are administered via IV or taken in pill form.

4. An (◯ expectorant, ◯ antitussive) is a drug to stimulate the production of saliva and induce coughing.

5. The primary ingredient in Sudafed is (◯ pseudoephedrine, ◯ phenylephrine).

UNIT 5
Using References

USING REFERENCES – INTRODUCTION

There was a lot of information in that last unit, and that the expectation is not that you know all of the drugs that are ever going to appear in a medical report. Naturally, there will be many that you will learn over time as you edit them often, but there are just too many drugs and they change too frequently to make it worthwhile to spend your time and energy memorizing them all up front.

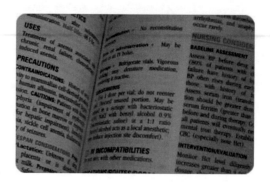

And the reality is that medications in medical reports pose some unique challenges for an MTE. Unlike symptoms listed under specific portions of the physical exam or instruments used during a particular surgical procedure, medications are generally not surrounded by sentence context. They are dictated primarily in lists. Brand-name medications also are difficult because they follow no rules, have no rhyme or reason to how they are spelled. And then there is navigating through all those dosage instructions. Furthermore, some dictators have been known to speed right through drug lists, slurring the medication name with the dose. That certainly doesn't make them any easier.

> While the Internet is a fantastic place to locate and verify drugs, it is a good idea to cross-reference the spelling of a drug using your program resources.

So, what happens when you are typing along and you hear a drug that you have never heard before? It will happen. And it will happen a lot. The Internet is a great place to locate drugs. In fact, it is such a good resource that most of your time in this unit will be spent introducing you to using it to the best possible advantage for finding medications.

This unit is full of online drug resource links and associated exercises. If you are unable to open a link for any reason (browser, firewall, etc), please know that you can use any reputable drug resource to complete the exercises on any given page.

ONLINE RESOURCES

There are an awful lot of resources for the pharmacology world. Luckily for you, many of them can be found right online. Of course, it may not be the best idea to just look up a drug on any old search engine—you never can tell where the information is coming from. Let's take a look at a few reputable online resources that can help you when you have questions about drugs.

EPOCRATES.COM

Epocrates.com is one of the best online resources to find reputable and accurate drug information. It is designed for and used by physicians but will be a great tool for you as well. You will need to sign up for a free account in order to use the site. When you sign up, choose Student as your occupation.

Epocrates provides a variety of tools and information. You can find drug information such as generic names, spelling, common dosages, and the purpose of the drug, as well as drug interactions, disease information, pill ID and pictures. Explore the site and see what else you can find. There are many features available to you with this resource. Not all will be used on the job but some may be useful in your everyday life as well.

The first medication in your list is Lipitor. Go to the website below and answer the following questions.

Create an account at online.epocrates.com and explore the site. Then use it to answer the questions below. Don't forget to look at the Drug Monograph list for addition information once you find the drug you are looking for.

Fill in the Blank.
Using the information on the given website, fill in the blanks.

1. The generic name of Lipitor is _____ .

2. Lipitor is prescribed to lower _____ .

3. Your doctor may prescribe Lipitor to reduce your chances of having a _____ .

4. The generic name of Lyrica is _____ .

5. Lyrica is prescribed to prevent or control _____ .

6. Your doctor may also prescribe Lyrica to treat pain caused by _____ damage.

Career Step is not affiliated with Epocrates.com. Epocrates.com is just one of many good sources available and is used here for illustrative purposes.

DRUGS.COM

Drugs.com is another website dedicated to drug information. According to their website, drugs.com is "the most popular, comprehensive and up-to-date source of drug information online. Providing free, peer-reviewed, accurate and independent advice on more than 24,000 prescription drugs, over-the-counter medicines and natural products."

Use the link to answer the questions.

On the main page, find the link for the "A-Z Drug List."

Multiple Choice.
Using the information on the given website, choose the best answer.

Click on the letter *D* and locate the drug term *Dalmane*.

1. Dalmane is used for _____.
   - ○ diabetes
   - ○ pain
   - ○ insomnia
   - ○ allergies

Without using the back button, go to the letter *M*, and locate the term *meclizine*.

2. What class of drug is meclizine?
   - ○ antidiabetic
   - ○ anticholinergic
   - ○ antidiuretic
   - ○ antianxiety

3. Which of the following is a trade name for meclizine?
   - ○ Antivert
   - ○ Dilantin
   - ○ Fosamax

Again, without using the back button, go to the letter *T*, and locate the term *Triamterene*.

4. Triamterene is a(n)
   - ○ anticholinergic
   - ○ diuretic
   - ○ beta blocker
   - ○ penicillin

It sounds like the dictator is saying "Toprol" and then a couple of letters.

5. Do a "drug search" on "Toprol." What are the missing letters?
   - ○ ST
   - ○ SL
   - ○ XL
   - ○ XT

Drugs.com has a number of features. Notice a list of "Featured Services" where you can find new drug approvals, new drug applications, alerts, a medical dictionary, forums, and mobile apps to name a few. Some of these services are also listed as links across the top. Spend some time clicking on the links and becoming familiar with the site and its features. It can be a great resource for you when you begin editing reports. Also notice a gray, rectangular box near the top of the page labeled "Medical Transcription." Click on it and see where you can use a wildcard and phonetic search to assist in identifying drugs. They also have a list of common drug misspellings. Career Step is not affiliated with Drugs.com or howjsay.com. Each is just one of many good sources available and is used here for illustrative purposes.

EXPRESS SCRIPTS

Another good basic online drug resource is provided by Express Scripts. You can find brand and generic names, forms the medication comes in, the drug type, the purpose of the drug and other information at this site.

Go to the Express Script to complete this exercise. Type the name of the medication in the search box and when the results page comes up, click on the drug name for detailed information.

Multiple Choice.
Using the information on the given website, choose the best answer.

1. The patient was prescribed Serevent to treat emphysema. What is the active ingredient in Serevent?
   - ○ bronchodilator
   - ○ salmeterol aerosol inhalation
   - ○ serevent
   - ○ albuterol

2. Actos is primarily used to treat which disease?
   - ○ glaucoma
   - ○ BPH
   - ○ type 2 diabetes
   - ○ hypertension

3. Search "lisinopril " and select one of the tablet options. Which of the following comes up as a representative (brand) name for the active ingredient (generic) "lisinopril?"
   - ○ Antivert
   - ○ Provera
   - ○ Zestril
   - ○ Lopid

4. You are pretty sure that the dictator says "dilantin," but you don't know if this is a generic drug or a brand name. Enter "dilantin" into the search window and determine if it is a brand name or a generic.
   - ○ brand name
   - ○ generic

Career Step is not affiliated with Express Scripts. This is just one of many good sources available and is used here for illustrative purposes.

FDA.GOV

FDA stands for Food and Drug Administration. This is the government organization in the United States responsible for approving and regulating prescription and nonprescription drugs. It is a veritable font of drug knowledge. Actually it is *the* font of drug knowledge. If a drug has been approved, it appears on this website.

There are actually several ways that you can use this website to get information about medications that may be dictated in medical reports you edit. Visit the site listed below and take a look at the home page for the FDA.

www.fda.gov

There is a lot of information here related to pretty much anything going on with the FDA. Foods. Drugs. Medical Devices. Biologics. Cosmetics. What is new in all of these areas. Their key initiatives. If you have an interest in all things food- and drug-related, this is definitely the place to be.

Of course, your interest is in drugs. From their main page, you can click on "Drugs," where you will find a wealth of additional information about all things drug-related. There are a couple of ways to effectively use this site, but all of them are better accessed at the following URL:

http://www.accessdata.fda.gov/scripts/cder/drugsatfda/index.cfm

Visit the site shown above. Notice that there are three different ways to find information about drugs from here.

- Search by Drug Name, Active Ingredient, or Application Number
- Browse by Drug Name
- Drug Approval Reports by Month

Depending on what information you are looking for, all of these can be useful tools. The **Search** tool on this site has a very cool feature that you will be working with a little bit later. But first, let's try a few exercises.

Multiple Choice.

Using the information on the given website, choose the best answer.

Let's find the drug metformin.

First, type the drug name into the Search feature.

By the sheer number of listings that comes up, you can be sure that you have it spelled correctly. Choose one of the brand name listings on the left hand side. Click into "Fortamet."

1. What dosage strength does this drug come in?

   ○ 100 mg

   ○ 200 mg

   ○ 500 mg

   ○ 800 mg

There is another way to look for metformin on this site. Go to the "M" in "Browse by Drug Name." Scroll down until you find metformin. (You will have to go to page 2.)

2. What is the full name of metformin?

   ○ metformin hydrochlorothiazide

   ○ metformin complete

   ○ metformin hydrochloride

   ○ metformin full strength

3. This drug is used for diabetes. Is it injected or in tablet form?

   ○ injected

   ○ tablet

Click into "Drug Approval Reports by Month." You can see that it allows you to choose a number of ways to (1.) select a report and (2.) select a month and year of the approval. Choose "All Approvals by Month" and "01/2008," and hit submit.

4. There was a new thyroid medication approved in January of 2008. Its active ingredient is levothyroxine sodium. What is the name of this drug?

   ○ Tirosint

   ○ Climara

   ○ Nutropin

   ○ Sular

5. A labeling revision for Lopressor is listed. Three actually. What is the active ingredient in Lopressor? (Also called the generic name.)

   ○ fentanyl

   ○ metformin

   ○ ibuprofen

   ○ metoprolol

WEBMD.COM

As you are starting to see, there are several different places that you can go to do some general research on looking up drugs. Another one is:

www.webmd.com

This site has a lot of general information about health and medicine. One of its specific features is a drug search, and there are a few different ways that you can look up drugs on this site. Let's go there now.

Go ahead and spend a few minutes looking around generally at what the site has to offer. Notice that there are tabs across the top. One of these is "Drugs & Supplements." Click on this link.

Like some of the other sites, it has a list of drugs by first letter. There are actually two different ways to look at drugs by first letter. The first tab (and the one which is default when you go to the site) is the Top 200 Drugs. Just to the right of that is Drugs A-Z. The pro of using the Top 200 Drugs is that it is a much smaller list, and therefore much easier to scan through. The con is, well, that it is a much smaller list, and therefore may not contain the drug that you are looking for.

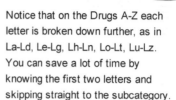

Highlights

Notice that on the Drugs A-Z each letter is broken down further, as in La-Ld, Le-Lg, Lh-Ln, Lo-Lt, Lu-Lz. You can save a lot of time by knowing the first two letters and skipping straight to the subcategory.

It doesn't really matter which one you look in, but let's practice looking up a few things.

Fill In The Blank.
Enter the correct words in the blanks provided.

1. Find the drug "Ativan" and click on it. This medication is used to treat _____ .

2. Find the drug nifedipine oral. This is used to treat angina (chest pain), and is sold under the brand name

   _____ .

3. Find the drug Omeprazole Oral. This drug blocks acid production in the stomach and is sold under the brand name

   _____ .

Multiple Choice.
Choose the best answer.

1. Find the drug Fumide Oral. Sold under the brand name Lasix, the correct generic term for this drug is:
   - ○ ferosemide
   - ○ furosemide
   - ○ furesomide
   - ○ ferusemide

Okay, now let's try to look up a drug by searching for it. Before we can do that, notice that on the Drugs & Supplements page there are actually two different search features. One is for all of WebMD; it is right next to the logo at the top. The other is more in the middle of the page and it is called Find A Drug. Technically, they will both work to look up drugs. The primary difference is that the Find a Drug feature looks only in the drug section—your results will look like they did when you found a drug by looking it up by first letter. In the main search feature, there will be a number of articles and additional information that will come up, including the "drug result." Both can be used to verify proper spelling and/or dosage information. Let's look at the difference.

First, type "glipizide" into the Find a Drug search. Make sure that you have selected the button "by name" and not "by condition."

A couple different listings come up, both are spelled "glipizide," both are oral tablets. Click on one of them. Read the first paragraph, and it will tell you what glipizide is used for. Or, notice at the bottom of the text box is a question, "What conditions does Glipizide Oral treat?"

Click on the question. It comes up:

Glipizide Oral is used to treat the following:
Type 2 Diabetes Mellitus

What if you knew that the drug the physician dictated was for type 2 diabetes mellitus, but you couldn't quite understand what he was saying. It sounded like it had a "p" sound and a "zide" sound. This time, do a search in the same place but use the "by condition" feature.

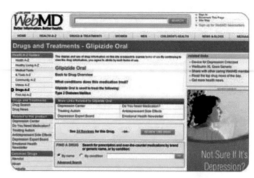

Two possibilities come up. Select the first one: Type 2 Diabetes Mellitus.

There it is, about a third of the way down, "glipizide." As an MTE, you can feel pretty confident that is what the dictator is saying. You know that it is used for the right condition, and it looks/sounds like what he was saying.

What happens if you put the drug into the general search feature? Go ahead and do that right now. It brings up several articles, many of which talk about diabetes mellitus in the heading or the brief description underneath the heading. You can be fairly certain at this point that a) you spelled it right and b) it's the right drug, as it is used for diabetes mellitus.

But what if you didn't know how to spell it for sure? Test it out. You know what it sounds like, but what is that initial sound?

Try putting in "clipizide." Whoa. Nothing came up, just one little question, "Did you mean: glipizide" and "glipizide" is a link. Click on it. There you are! All the information that you need, and you can be pretty sure it's spelled right now.

Try typing in "glipazide." What happens?

How about "glupizide?"

You see, as long as you're close, it brings up the right medication. Now you try a few. Click on the following links, listen to the drug, and find it using any method you want to on this site.

GENERAL LOOK-UPS

The previous sites are all great for looking up drugs. There are also websites that incorporate some of the above focused drug sites along with other types of searches. These could be searches of online dictionaries, abbreviations, ICD codes, and even hospitals or doctors in specific hospitals. Since drugs will undoubtedly not be the only thing you spend some time researching, you may want to familiarize yourself with a few of these sites, and practice looking up some drugs from them.

First, let's go to:

www.mt911.com

On the main page, there is a list of the different search engines and listings available. For drugs, you want to click on "Drug names." (That should be pretty obvious.) Read the directions and decide which search you want to use and find the following medications.

Career Step is not affiliated with mt911.com, scribera.net, or medilexicon.com. These are just some of the many good sources available and are used here for illustrative purposes.

IT ALL LOOKS A LITTLE FUZZY

What do we mean by fuzzy? This is not the same type of fuzzy you would use to describe your favorite teddy bear. This is, however, the same type of fuzzy you would use to describe your vision before you put your glasses on in the morning. But what do these descriptive definitions of fuzzy have to do with finding a medication?

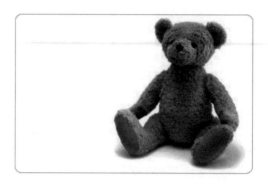

Let's say that you have a vague idea of the word you are looking for, but you are not quite sure you can figure out all of the letters—or even most of the letters. The dictator is speaking very fast or the dictation cuts out in the middle of the word. Back in my day, there really wasn't a lot that you could do. Hours in various drug books. But even that wasn't particularly helpful if the first part of the word was cut off—where do you even begin? But today, with the Internet, there are amazing search engines that give you the option to do a "fuzzy" search—a search that looks for the bits and pieces of the word that you give it in any place within the word.

As you go with a fuzzy idea of a word in mind to one of the sites outlined earlier in this unit, be sure to read any instructions that the sites provide so that you can make the most of their features. Some sites may allow you to perform fuzzy searches using an asterisk, while others may require you use a different symbol or no symbol at all.

A great site for fuzzy medication searches is one you have been to before. I told you that we would be coming back to it. And here it is.

http://www.accessdata.fda.gov/scripts/cder/drugsatfda/index.cfm?fuseaction=Search.Search_Drug_Name

Drugs@FDA allows you to perform a fuzzy search using a minimum of only 3 consecutive characters. The results will show the letters you used in bold within the medication. The group of letters can occur at the beginning, end, or even the middle of the word! The results this site gives will include both drug names and active ingredients—what a treat!

Let's practice using it. Visit the site listed above.

First, let's get an idea of how this works. The drug is Allegra. Type the three letters at the end ("gra") into the first search option: "Search by Drug Name, Active Ingredient, or Application Number." There it is! Third from the top. Try the first three letters ("All-"). Yup. A little further down, but still there. How about the middle letters ("leg."). What do you know? It came up first!

Multiple Choice.
Using the information on the given website, choose the best answer.

1. The dictation is cut off. It sounds like maybe a long "O" sound and it ends in "vask" or "vasc." Say it out loud, so you get an idea of what it sounded like. Then type the two strings of 4 letters into the search box and take an educated guess on what the correct medication might be.

   ○ Norvasc

   ○ Univasc

   ○ Vascor

   ○ Iprivask

Fill In The Blank.
Enter the correct word in the blank provided.

1. The beginning of the word is cut off. End sounds like "vacid" or "vasid." Enter the drug you think it is based on the search results.

   _____

2. The dictator is speaking really fast. The only thing you're pretty sure of is in the middle of the word, and it sounds like "soap-ra." Try whatever combination of letters you think that may be. What drug is it likely to be?_____

3. It seems clear that the initial sound of the drug is an "f" sound. You are not sure if it will start with "f" or "ph." The end of the drug sounds like "ode-a-peen." What drug is it likely to be?_____

4. It sounds for all the world like the dictator is saying "Norman" is the drug. But the initial sound may be cut off. What do you think the drug is?_____(HINT: Go ahead and try "Norman." Nothing comes up. What is another way you could spell what sounds like "Norman?" If you change out that last vowel, "normen," "normin," "normon," and "normun," it really makes this one easy!)

KNOW THE DOSE

Medications are always prescribed at a specific dose—the amount of the medicine that the physician thinks will help the patient. And while the dose can be a tricky part of editing medications, it is also another clue. And the clues work both ways. Sometimes knowing the dose can help you find the right medication, and sometimes knowing the right medication can help you find the right dose.

Depending on how fast or garbled the dictator is, numbers can be wonderfully familiar amidst a minefield of mushed sounds. Especially when those mushed sounds are meant to be medications but sound more like pig Latin than English. You may have occasions where you cannot, for the life of you, pick out the name of the medicine, but you can clearly understand the dose that follows it. If that's the case, there are sites that allow you to search by dose.

If this link does not work for you for any reason, please feel free to use any reputable drug resource to complete the exercises on this page.

One such site is http://pennmedicine.adam.com/content.aspx?productId=46
(This page is entitled "Drug Interactions" but it is the correct page for this type of search. Simply go to box #1 and type in the dosage.)

One thing to be aware of is that, when searching by dose only, you can enter only the number, not the unit of measure. And the results will include all the medications with that number anywhere in the dose. For instance, if you search for "80," the results will include medications that come in "800" and "580" and so on. Obviously, you have to have some vague notion of what the medication sounds like so you can see if there are any that seem to match. While this may seem daunting, it sure is easier than trying to find a drug by a specific dose in a pharmaceutical wordbook. I promise!

Let's try a few.

Fill in the Blank.
Using the information on the given website, enter the correct word in the blanks provided.

1. All you can tell for sure is that the first letter is "z." It may have an "a" after it, but you aren't certain. You can hear the dosage perfectly clear. 150 b.i.d. Can you find any medication that you think may work? _____

2. Here's another one; he's just speaking so fast. The initial sound is probably an "r" and there is definitely a "t" and an "n" somewhere in it. But the dosage is 75 mg. Of that you are certain. Can you find a drug that may fit the bill? _____

So how do dosages work the other way? Well, if you can clearly hear the medication but you're not so sure about the dose, many of the sites have dosage information available with the drug information. Obviously, a dose of 25 mg is very different from 2.5 mg. And the difference between a gram and a milligram is huge, so it's very important that you edit the correct one. For the exercise below, you'll need to use a different website or your drug reference to find the correct dose.

Multiple Choice.
Choose the best answer.

1. The patient is on hydrochlorothiazide (2.5 mg, 25 mg).
2. She was prescribed fludrocortisone (0.1 mg, 1 mg).
3. And for pain, Tramadol (50 mg, 500 mg).

Career Step is not affiliated with the University of Pennsylvania. The University of Pennsylvania Drug Interactions tool is just one of many good sources available and is used here for illustrative purposes.

THE RIGHT CONDITION

Sometimes knowing what medical condition the drug is being prescribed for can be a tremendous help in locating the right medication. Unfortunately, medications are often part of a list that does not have any context...it's just a list. However, you can look for clues about the patient's conditions in the rest of the report. You can try looking at any past medical history provided, the admission or discharge diagnosis, other reasons mentioned in the body of a report (such as pain control after a procedure), or any other condition mentioned in the report. All this searching for clues, are you starting to feel like a character in a *National Treasure* movie?

If you can't figure out the medication, http://www.drugs.com/medical_conditions.html has a feature on its site that allows you to search by condition. Popular conditions are listed in plain view, while other conditions can be searched for by using their alphabetical listing located immediately below the most popular conditions list.

Give it a try. Visit the site. This is a site you have been to before, but last time you were at the tab "Drugs & Medications." This time you are at "Diseases & Conditions." You can go directly to Drugs.com and click on the tab, or you can click on the link above and it will take you to "Diseases & Conditions." You are looking for a medication for cholesterol. Click on cholesterol on the main part of the page.

Scroll down through the page until you get to the list of the 20 most popular drugs used to treat high cholesterol. Chances are pretty good that if you were looking for a drug you knew was prescribed to lower cholesterol, it would appear on that list.

You may remember that another site we worked on had a drug search feature specifically by condition. That website is:

www.WebMD.com

Career Step is not affiliated with WebMD.com. WebMD.com is just one of many good sources available and is used here for illustrative purposes.

THAT FABULOUS FIND FEATURE

Before we get too far away from enjoying these long lists of conditions and drugs, we want to point out a great feature that you have in your browser that you may not even be aware of: **find**. Quite apart from the Internet, it works as part of your browser on the page that you have open.

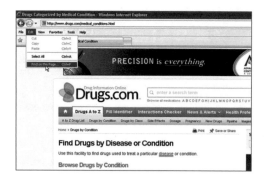
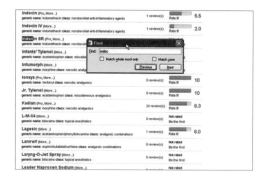

You can see how your browser's **find** feature can come in quite handy when trying to search through a seemingly never-ending list, such as the list you'll encounter if you search under the condition "Pain" on drugs.com.

Try using it. Go to www.drugs.com/medical_conditions.html

Click on "Pain." Using the **find** feature on your browser (usually control + F), slowly type the following pieces of drug terms, one letter at a time. Notice when the drug to the right comes up, highlighting the characters that you have typed. (Of note, this will work differently depending on your browser.)

1. o-x-y-c→OxyContin
2. l-o-r-t→Lortab
3. p-e-r-c→Percocet
4. v-i-c→Vicodin
5. l-a-u→Dilaudid

Isn't that cool? It is certainly faster and easier than scanning a big long list, especially if you are unclear on the initial sound. Working much the same as a "fuzzy" search, it works on any webpage that contains the whole list within it and can be a great timesaver when it comes to researching drugs.

Career Step is not affiliated with Drugs.com. Drugs.com is just one of many good sources available and is used here for illustrative purposes.

SOUNDS LIKE, BUT NOT QUITE

Although you can't relate to it yet, you will someday have one (or probably more) of those moments when the dictator says something and you find a word that matches. Or it could match...it almost matches...except for *one little, itty-bitty thing*. As much as you want to type it in that way and move on, you have a nagging feeling, a tapping on the inside of your skull, saying, "Excuse me. Excuse me! That's just not quite right." As much as you want it to be the right term, you just know that it isn't. But it's *so close...*

Sometimes medications (as well as other medical terms) sound so similar it can be dangerous. Some of the websites we've introduced you to, as well as your pharmaceutical wordbook or software, include a feature that indicates "sound-alike" medications. These are meds that either written or spoken are similar enough that they can easily be confused for each other.

Keep in mind that they might not seem particularly similar when looking at them, but they might sound very similar when dictated, especially by a doctor with a mouth full of marbles. (We haven't yet figured out why doctors fill their mouths with marbles. It must have something to do with the great mystique of knowledge...) If you have any doubts whatsoever, it can't hurt to do a quick check to see if the medication you think you hear has an evil twin (or another option), but it might hurt not to. Use one of your many reputable drug resources to identify the following medications.

Don't let this section discourage you. Most dictators really do speak clearly enough that you can tell the difference, even between terms that are this similar. And for the ones that don't, there is usually enough of a clue in the context that you can figure it out. But even if worse comes to worst, you can flag it to the attention of the client. They will recognize you for the incredibly talented and diligent medical transcription editor that you are, and be grateful for the feedback.

TO CAPITALIZE OR NOT, THAT IS THE QUESTION

You know the difference between brand name and generic medications. But even so, perhaps one of the most frequent questions students have about medications is still when to capitalize them. You may have noticed by now that many drug sites capitalize ALL medications, some even using capital letters for the entire name! This certainly doesn't help clear up the confusion. Make sure that you take note of this when you're searching a medication site. You should be able to pretty quickly determine which ones fall into this category so that you know if it's one that you can rely on for proper capitalization.

> **ONE SIMPLE RULE:**
> Capitalize brand names and don't capitalize generic names.

The inconsistency in these sites feeds the notion that there is no real method to the capitalization madness, but it really is just one simple rule: capitalize brand names and don't capitalize generic names.

Of course, like any rule, even a simple one, there is an exception. Always capitalize any word that begins a sentence, and for that matter, a numbered list in a medical report. It's the redeeming feature of those long medication lists—every drug tends to be capitalized and you don't have to expend the time and energy looking up whether it's generic or brand name.

This is what a numbered medication list looks like.

Medical Record

DISCHARGE MEDICATIONS

1. Coumadin 5 mg p.o. q.d.
2. Enalapril 2.5 mg p.o. q.d.
3. Cardizem SR 90 mg b.i.d.
4. Mevacor 20 mg q.d.
5. Lopressor 20 mg b.i.d.
6. Nitroglycerin sublingual p.r.n. q.5 minutes times 3 for chest pain.

DISCHARGE MEDICATIONS

1. Cephradine 250 mg one tablet p.o. t.i.d. times ten days.
2. Ferrous sulfate 325 mg one tablet p.o. t.i.d.
3. Aspirin, enteric-coated 325 mg one tablet p.o. q. daily.
4. Chlorpromazine 25 mg one tablet q.12 hours.
5. Darvocet-N 100 1-2 tablets q.3 hours p.r.n. pain.
6. Docusate sodium 240 mg one tablet p.o. b.i.d.
7. Famotidine 20 mg one tablet p.o. b.i.d.
8. Lovastatin 20 mg one tablet p.o. h.s.

WHAT IS YOUR SPECIALTY?

There is yet another way to search for a medication when you have a good idea of what condition it is being prescribed for, and that is to search according to specialty. On the Internet there are many sites focused on one particular specialty, listing all sorts of things related to that specialty, including medications. The advantage of this type of search is that you don't have to wade through long lists of unrelated medications. The disadvantage is that you may have to go to more than one site looking for an easy-to-read and pertinent list of drugs for a given specialty. Probably not your first option when researching drugs, it is still useful to know and practice. (Especially if you get stuck in an obscure specialty, or one you rarely work on, and find it mostly unfamiliar.)

So, how do you find specialty sites? To search for such sites, simply go to www.google.com and search for [specialty] + medications. You would insert the specialty you are looking for inside the brackets. A search for cardiology medications would look like this in the Google search box: cardiology + medications. You can type it with spaces on either side of the + sign or without them; it makes no difference whatsoever.

So, if you were looking for chemotherapy medications, you would type chemotherapy + medications in a Google box. One of the first, if not the first, sites that comes up is

http://www.chemocare.com/bio

Visit the link listed above. You can see a rather succinct list of several chemotherapy drugs.

Again, this is probably a last-resort kind of search, when all of your tried and true sites fail you and you're still researching...

WOULD YOU LIKE SOME HERBS WITH THAT?

Occasionally you'll find that a patient is taking herbs or supplements. Actually, patients will frequently be taking herbs and supplements but only occasionally will they be reported in the patient's medication information. Herbs sometimes have unusual names, so this can leave an MT wondering if they really just heard the doctor say that the patient is taking Crazy Apple and Yerba Santa—surely I have been sitting here and typing a little too long and he must have said something else!

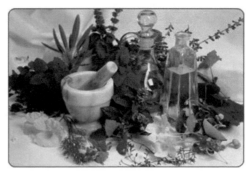

Well, just like there are great medication sites for prescription and over-the-counter drug searches, there are great herb and supplement sites for herb and supplement searches. http://www.drugdigest.org is just such a site, even providing information such as scientific name, other names, and uses.

NOTE: This website is down at the present time, so please go to http://www.drugs.com to complete this exercise. Hover your mouse over the Drugs A-Z tab and select "Natural Products" from the menu. You will then see an A-Z Index. Use this to select the herb in order to answer the questions below.

Multiple Choice.
Using information from the website given, choose the best answer.

1. Find "ginkgo." Which of the following is not another name for "ginkgo"?

   ○ Japanese Silver Apricot

   ○ Mythical Bush

   ○ Kew Tree

   ○ Maidenhair Tree

2. Butcher's Broom is the active ingredient in topical treatments for which of the following conditions?

   ○ acne

   ○ hemorrhoids

   ○ folliculitis

   ○ shingles

3. What is the scientific name for "Witch Hazel"?

   ○ Centella asiatica

   ○ Tabebuia avellanedae

   ○ Hamamelis viginiana

   ○ Apis mellifera

Career Step is not affiliated with drugdigest.org or drugs.com. They are just some of many good sources available and is used here for illustrative purposes.

GOING STRAIGHT TO THE HORSE'S MOUTH

One of the wonderful things about the Internet is the staggering volume of information available on it. Pretty much every company that sells anything wants as much information about what they sell available to the public. And drug companies are no exception. Think about it. When a new drug comes out, it's advertised on TV! You are urged to talk to your doctor about drugs when you have no idea what they are for or why you would possibly want them. Believe it or not, there is actually something good about that—all that information on all those drugs is available in colorful marketing websites.

Information that can be found at a drug company website:

- what a drug is used for
- the generic name
- what form it comes in
- dosages it is manufactured in
- who manufactures it

You can quickly and easily find a lot of information by going directly to the website dedicated to that brand-name drug. A key word here is *brand-name*. There are no pretty marketing websites for generic drugs or drug ingredients. But when looking for information on a brand-name drug, it is sometimes the best source there is.

Look at the following example.

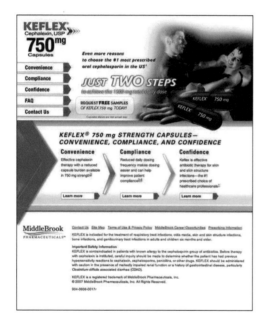

With just a few clicks and by looking at the home page of this drug (Keflex), you can see:

- the generic drug is cephalexin
- it is a cephalosporin (a group of antibiotics)
- it comes in 750 mg doses
- it is a capsule
- it is an antibiotic
- it is used to treat:
-
  - respiratory tract infections
  - otitis media (ear infections)
  - skin and skin structure infections
  - bone infections
  - genitourinary tract infections
- as of 2006 it is on the market
- it is made by MiddleBrook Pharmaceuticals

There are lots of ways that this can be useful. You can verify what it's used for, what the dosages are, any letters or numbers that may be part of the prescribed drug name. In fact, there is enough information on one of these websites that you can be very confident, with very little context, that you have the right drug, it's spelled right, and you have the right dosage.

Another nice thing about these sites is that they often come up first or second in a search. How do you know which sites they are? Generally speaking, the name of the drug itself is the web address, such as www.coumadin.com and www.humalog.com or contains the name of the drug company in the web address or lists "products," such as http://www.roche.com/products-us.htm.

You can eliminate web addresses that come up that you know by now, like www.drugs.com/valium.html. This is the web address for the description of Valium found on www.drugs.com.

You try a few…

Find the website for the drug Humalog. (Type it in a search engine box, like Google.) Look at that! It's right at the top, www.humalog.com

By the way, if you spelled Humalog wrong, the search engine will often catch it and ask if you meant the right spelling. Try that. Type Humulog instead of Humalog and see what happens.

Multiple Choice.
Choose the best answer.

1. Humalog is a brand name _____.
   - ○ antibiotic
   - ○ calcium channel blocker
   - ○ insulin
   - ○ anesthetic

2. Humalog comes with a fancy delivery system called _____.
   - ○ quick pen
   - ○ InsulinIsFun
   - ○ KwikPen
   - ○ Kwikpen

Now let's take a look at Lipitor. This one is easy, as it even says, in big bold letters "Official Site!"

3. What is the #1 reason that Lipitor is prescribed?
   - ○ chest pain
   - ○ lower cholesterol
   - ○ support patients
   - ○ control blood sugar

4. What is the generic name for Lipitor?
   - ○ atorvastatin calcium
   - ○ fluvastatin
   - ○ simvastatin

Career Step is not affiliated with MiddleBrook Pharmaceuticals, Bristol-Myers Squibb Company, Eli Lilly and Company, or Roche Pharmaceuticals. These are just some of the many good sources available and are used here for illustrative purposes.

SAY WHAT?!

Every now and then you might find that a medication and/or dose causes a little red flag to appear in your mind. Just like any other item in a medical report, a dictator can (and will) make a mistake while dictating medications—the wrong medication, the wrong dosage, the wrong measurement. It's not necessarily your responsibility as an MTE to catch a mistake in dosage or medication, but doing so will make you that much more valuable to your client. And sometimes just asking them to verify that something is correct can help solidify your value to the integrity of the record in the mind of the client or the physician.

For the most part, as you edit the same dictators and the same types of reports over time, you will become familiar enough with the parameters of medications and their uses that you will have red flags shoot up all on their own. In the meantime, there are a few things that you can look out for.

> The patient was sent home with a prescription for 800 gm ibuprofen p.r.n. pain.

This should sound some alarm bells.

MEDICAL RECORD

HISTORY: This is a seven-year-old female who was swimming and slipped on the edge of the pool. She said she hit her chin, which started bleeding. Denied any loss of consciousness. She has no headache, no blurred vision, slurred speech, no nausea or vomiting.

PHYSICAL EXAMINATION: Shows a very pleasant female in no acute distress. Temperature 97.4, pulse 80, respirations 20, blood pressure 110/68. HEENT: benign, pupils PERRLA, EOMs intact; discs are flat and sharp. She has a 3 cm laceration to her chin, which was actively bleeding.

Vigorous irrigation with normal saline and Betadine was performed. 2% lidocaine was used to anesthetize the area with good results. A running stitch of 3-0 Ethilon was performed without any complications.

IMPRESSION: 3 cm laceration to the chin.

PLAN: Patient education on wound care was given to the mother. Followup in 2 days for wound check, 8-10 days to have suture removal, sooner if her mother notices any signs of infection, redness, swelling, pus, or any other problems. She was given a prescription for Glucophage 500 mg for pain.

Even with the little exposure you have had thus far to medications, you may remember that Glucophage is an antidiabetic drug. A seven-year-old girl in for stitches probably doesn't need a diabetic medication, especially not for pain. Of course, as an MTE you have no possible way of knowing what the real medication is. Although you could take an educated guess, you would never ever do that. You would need to put a note on the report so that the physician could verify and add the proper drug.

In some instances, however, what he said is exactly what he meant. There are some medications that can be used outside of their usual purpose. For example, very high doses of a corticosteroid such as prednisone can be given as short-term therapy for autoimmune hemolytic anemia. The upshot is that you can't be sure, but you should trust your instincts. Always flag things you are not sure of.

You also might find that a little bit of extra research puts together pieces of the puzzle that had you stumped. You can do this extra research by using a search engine, such as www.google.com and multiple key words for your search. Take the instance of a high dose of a corticosteroid. You might have enough information in the report to search for 'corticosteroid + "high dose" + "autoimmune hemolytic anemia"' and find that, yes, in fact, corticosteroids are administered in high doses to patients with autoimmune hemolytic anemia.

In the following exercises, determine if anything seems out of the ordinary or sends up a red flag, and if so, what. Use any and all resources that we've discussed so far, but do the research. Look up everything and make sure it's right. Normally, you wouldn't need to verify *everything* in your medications list, but this is good practice for looking things up.

Multiple Choice.
Determine whether the following prescriptions should be flagged or not.

1. Current Medications:

   1. Felodipine for knee pain. 2. Cetirizine for sinus symptoms. 3. Aspirin daily.

   ○ Flag it

   ○ It's fine

2. She was prescribed metformin for polycystic ovarian disease.

   ○ Flag it

   ○ It's fine

3. The patient was prescribed Coumadin 75 mg.

   ○ Flag it

   ○ It's fine

4. Toprol-XL 5000 mg a day was prescribed for high blood pressure.

   ○ Flag it

   ○ It's fine

5. She has been taking 5000 mg of a garlic supplement.

   ○ Flag it

   ○ It's fine

OUT WITH THE OLD, IN WITH THE NEW

While you may not be interested in owning the latest Hummer or having a cell phone that can take pictures, play music, and work as an actual phone all at the same time, you will most likely be interested in always having the most up-to-date drug list at your fingertips. Prescriptions are always changing, and even for the latest pharmaceutical references, this can present a small problem with effectively searching for medications. It might be beneficial to keep track of new medications that you find and verify online by scribbling them in any reference book or tool you keep within arm's length at all times.

Breaking medication news can be found on a number of sites. A couple of these include:
http://www.accessdata.fda.gov/scripts/cder/drugsatfda/index.cfm?fuseaction=Reports.ReportsMenu and http://www.prescribingreference.com

Take a moment now to go check them out, recognizing that medication news is just that—NEW—and it's changing all the time. One of these sites is the FDA site you have been to before, but the other one is new. You can also put "medication news" into a search engine and see what other sites have the latest and greatest information.

A WORD ABOUT HOMELAND "SURETY"

Whenever looking for medication information, always be sure to select information pertinent to the *country* you are typing reports for. This is especially important when dealing with drugs, because drugs often have different names based totally on the country they are distributed in. For example, the common antinausea medication Dramamine is sold in Canada under the name Gravol.

You can often determine the country of origin of a site by looking at the web address.

If the address includes ".ca" then it is for Canada. For example, the site for Gravol is found at

gravol.ca/

If the address includes ".uk" then it is for the United Kingdom. The generic drug sertraline is sold in the United States under the brand name Zoloft and in the United Kingdom as Lustral. Note the following website and the presence of ".uk" in it.

www.netdoctor.co.uk/medicines/100001555.html

If the address includes ".au" then it is for Australia. What is sold in the United States as Tylenol is sold in Australia (and the United Kingdom for that matter) as Panadol. A good general medication site based in Australia is

www.mydr.com.au/search/cmi

Of course, there are many others, largely in languages other than English. Because of this, they probably won't come up all that often as you are doing medical transcription editing.

Keep in mind that addresses do not always indicate what country the information is intended for. And when it comes to drugs, the country can have a lot to do with the right drug. If you are uncertain whether the site you are looking at is based in the right country, take a look around and see if it provides any other information that might indicate location, such as an address or telephone number.

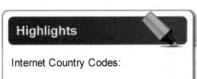

Highlights

Internet Country Codes:

- .uk (United Kingdom)
- .au (Australia)
- .nz (New Zealand)
- .ca (Canada)
- .il (Israel)
- .za (South Africa)
- .ph (Philippines)
- .in (India)

UNIT 6

Formatting

FORMATTING – INTRODUCTION

You may think that now that you have learned all about how drugs are administered, been exposed to several drug categories—as well as numerous individual drug names—and you are confident that you will be able to find anything you hear, you are pretty much finished with medications. You may think so and then the first time you heard a drug list dictated you would be very, very sad. What on earth is the dictator saying after the drug name?!? Numbers, letters, numbers and letters, all jumbled together. You never dreamed that getting the drug name would be the easy part!

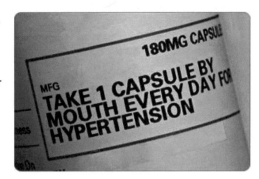

It should come as no surprise that physicians don't just hand out various drugs to their patients and hope it all works out. Drugs are prescribed in specific amounts with specific instructions. Generally, the amount of medicine to be given at any one time is called a dose and the total amount of doses administered is called the dosage. However, different doctors (and even dictionaries) often use the terms interchangeably.

In any case, what it means to you as an MTE is that you will often have a drug dictated immediately followed by dosage instructions. These instructions can include all or some of the following:

- the size or amount of medication to be given
- the frequency with which it should be taken
- when it should be taken
- how and/or where it should be taken
- the total number of doses (or pills)
- the duration or course of the treatment

That sounds great, but what does it look like? Let me give you a few examples.

TOPROL XL 50 MG 1 P.O. Q. DAY

- In this example there is the name of the medication: Toprol XL
- the size or amount: 50 mg
- the frequency: 1 q. day (1 per day)
- how or where it should be taken: p.o. (by mouth)

CLARITHROMYCIN 500 MG P.O. B.I.D. X 8 D. TO COMPLETE COURSE OF 10 DAYS.

- name: Clarithromycin
- amount: 500 mg
- frequency: b.i.d. (twice a day)
- how: p.o. (by mouth)
- duration: 10 day course

FUROSEMIDE P.R.N.

- name: furosemide
- frequency: p.r.n. (as needed)

That's it! No other information at all. One important thing to remember is that a dictator may give you nothing but the name of the medication, the name and one piece of information, some of the above information, or tell you everything you could ever want to know about that medication and when/how/for how long it gets into that patient. You will only be able to edit what he/she dictates.

Of course, like anything else with medical transcription editing, the more you know about how medicines are given, the easier this will be when you begin your work. So, let's take each of these in a lot more detail.

UNITS OF MEASUREMENT

The modern form of the "metric system" is called the International System of Units (SI). It was actually adopted internationally in 1960, including by the United States! It is also not a static system—units are created and definitions modified through an international agreement. With the exception of the U.S., most countries do not even have official definitions of any other standard of measurement. Medicine (and science) overwhelmingly employs this measuring system. And for you that means dosages!

For those who are not familiar with the metric system, let's break it down as simply as possible.

The metric system is based on the number 10. Unlike pounds (which are 16 ounces) or feet (which are 12 inches), everything in SI somehow related to the number 10. For the purposes of pharmacology, let's start with a gram (g) which is a thousandth of a kilogram (kg). That's not very much—about 1/28 of an ounce. Why talk about a kilogram in this module at all? Your body weight is measured in kilograms, so obviously your medication never ever will be. However, it may be helpful to know that a kilogram is considered the base unit of mass in SI. What is mass? The mass of an object is often referred to as its weight, and it is how many drugs are measured.

Let's keep breaking it down. A milligram (mg) is an order of magnitude less than a gram. It is a thousandth of a gram to be precise—a very small quantity indeed.

Finally, a microgram is a thousandth of a milligram—or one millionth of a gram—a really, really small quantity. This term is technically abbreviated µg, but for transcription editing purposes it is much easier and more commonly represented as mcg, so you don't need to worry about finding a special character.

Using a kilogram as the base unit of mass, let's look at 1 kilogram and how much that is in g, mg, and mcg.

kilogram – 1

gram – 1000*

milligram – 1,000,000

microgram – 1,000,000,000

*note-when editing numbers with four numerals, such as 1000, it can be edited with or without a comma (1000 or 1,000). Your account instructions may specify which is preferred.

You can look at it another way too. If you have 1 gram, how much is that in kg, mg, and mcg?

kilogram – 1/1000

gram – 1

milligram – 1000

microgram – 1,000,000

By far the most common unit of measurement in medication is the milligram (mg), although micrograms and even grams are sometimes used. And you can imagine the importance of not getting these mixed up. You would be off by a factor of a thousand. Give a thousand times too little, and a drug probably won't do much of anything; give a thousand times too much, and it might very well kill the patient.

Another term specific to pharmacology is the International Unit (IU). This is based on measuring the biological activity or the effect of a substance. It is used for vitamins, hormones, some drugs, vaccines, and blood products. It is not part of the SI. You don't really need to know how it works, just that it exists and you will see it in medical reports. It is usually abbreviated, and as rule #2 below shows, should be abbreviated even if it is dictated as "international unit."

As far as using these terms in medical reports, you should know a couple of rules.

1. Never abbreviate a term that a doctor dictates in full except for units of measurements: mg, mcg, cm, mm.
2. When editing units of measurement, use the Arabic numeral and abbreviate the measurement.

CORRECT: 5 mg, 10 mm, 150 mg
INCORRECT: 5 milligrams, ten mm, a hundred and fifty milligrams

Let's make sure that you're comfortable with these very common units of measurements and basic rules about using them before going on.

Fill in the Blank.
Expand or abbreviate the letters/word in the blank provided.

1. g   _____

2. gram   _____

3. kg   _____

4. kilogram   _____

5. mg   _____

6. milligram   _____

7. mcg   _____

8. microgram   _____

9. IU   _____

10. International Unit   _____

Matching.
Match the appropriate terms below.

1. ____ µg   A. International Unit

2. ____ g   B. kilogram

3. ____ IU   C. microgram

4. ____ mg   D. gram

5. ____ kg   E. milligram

Multiple Choice.
Choose the best answer.

1. The SI or International System of Units uses _____.

   ○ base 100

   ○ base 20

   ○ base 16

   ○ base 10

2. If a physician prescribes a patient one hundred milligrams of a drug, you would edit this _____.

   ○ 100 mcg

   ○ 100 mg

   ○ one hundred milligrams

   ○ 1000 mcg

3. You should abbreviate a word that a dictator states in full _____.

   ○ never

   ○ always

   ○ only in units of measurement

4. If something weighs 12 g, it is how many milligrams?

   ○ 12

   ○ 1,200

   ○ 12,000

   ○ 12,000,000

5. The mass of most drugs is calculated in _____.

   ○ ounces

   ○ milligrams

   ○ kilograms

   ○ pounds

THE METRIC SYSTEM

Sometimes drugs are not measured in terms of mass but in terms of *volume*. And volume is measured a little differently. Since you are not a pharmacist, and don't need to be, all of the nuances and chemical formulas are not really important. But there are a few things you should know.

A **liter**, abbreviated **L** or **l** and spelled litre outside the United States, is an amount slightly more than a quart in the U.S. Drugs are not typically measured in liters, although they can be inserted into liters of fluid and administered intravenously. Additionally, in medical reports urine output is sometimes measured in liters.

For purposes of pharmacology, the **milliliter**, abbreviated **mL** or **ml** and spelled millilitre outside of the U.S., is much more common. A milliliter is 1/1000 of a liter and is frequently represented as a **cubic centimeter** or **cc**, the two being equivalent. (1 cc=1 mL)

Another term used specifically in chemistry and the biological sciences is called an equivalent (Eq). Basically it is a measure of a substance's ability to combine with other substances. In the field of medical transcription, the amount of a pharmacological substance is small enough to be measured not in equivalents, but in *milliequivalents (mEq)*. Of course, by now you have seen *milli-* enough that you probably know this means 1/1000 of an equivalent. As with grams and milligrams, a dictator will generally say the whole term, as in "milliequivalents," and you will transcribe it as "mEq."

Another common unit of measurement is the **calorie**. In the SI system, the calorie has largely been replaced by the term **joule**, although you will see both terms in medical reports. Even more frequently, however, you will see a **kilocalorie**, which is abbreviated **kcal** in medical reports.

Fill in the Blank.
Retype the term in the blank provided.

1. L or l   _____

2. liter   _____

3. mL or ml   _____

4. milliliter   _____

5. cc   _____

6. cubic centimeter _____

7. mEq   _____

8. milliequivalents _____

9. calorie   _____

10. kcal   _____

11. kilocalorie   _____

Fill in the Blank.

The following abbreviations and terms are taught on this page. Fill in the appropriate blank with either the abbreviation or its expansion.

1. mEq   _____

2. cc   _____

3. liter   _____

4. milliliter   _____

5. kilocalorie   _____

6. L   _____

7. kcal   _____

8. mL   _____

9. milliequivalents   _____

10. cubic centimeter   _____

MEASURING UP IN THE USA

Although the International System of Units is predominantly used for dosing drugs, if you are editing in the United States, chances are pretty good that you will type units of measurement that are NOT SI. Americans buy milk and fill baby bottles using ounces, and they cook in pounds, teaspoons, and tablespoons. There are just a few that we are going to review here.

First is the **ounce**, abbreviated **oz**. Unlike systems that use base 10, the ounce is, well, sort of an arbitrary amount as far as international recognition goes. So, purely for curiosity sake, an ounce is 28.349523 grams. At least an ounce in the United States is that much. A Troy ounce, which used to be common in the United Kingdom is 31.1034768 grams. Whether by volume or mass it is the same, except by volume we call it a **fluid ounce**. This is abbreviated **fl oz**.

The **pound** is another Americanism. At least as it regards to weight. In Great Britain, the pound refers to money (based on a pound mass of silver). In the United States a pound is equal to 16 oz and it is abbreviated **lb** (**lbs** for "pounds"). In medical reports, you really won't ever see anyone prescribed a pound of medicine. You will see this frequently, however, in regards to the patient's weight, so it's useful to know.

Liquid medicine is sometimes prescribed by the **teaspoon** or tablespoon and both are considered units of volume, although in pharmacology the teaspoon is far more common. It is abbreviated **tsp** and by volume is approximately equivalent to 5 mL. A tablespoon (tbs) is approximately 3 teaspoons, and as far as most medicines go, would be quite a lot.

Fill in the Blank.
Retype the abbreviation or term in the blank provided.

1. oz   _____

2. ounce   _____

3. fl oz   _____

4. fluid ounce   _____

5. lb   _____

6. pound   _____

7. tsp   _____

8. teaspoon   _____

Fill in the Blank.
The following abbreviations and terms are taught on this page. Fill in the appropriate blank with either the abbreviation or its expansion.

1. lb   _____

2. fluid ounce   _____

3. tsp   _____

4. pound   _____

5. oz   _____

6. ounce   _____

7. fl oz   _____

8. teaspoon   _____

PER-PER-PERFECT ZERO

Sometimes, especially if a patient is admitted to the hospital and receiving drugs intravenously, drug doses are expressed in relation to the weight of the patient. A dictator would say, for example, the name of the drug and "five milligrams per kilogram." That means that the patient is given a dose equal to 5 mg for each kilogram that the patient weighs. So, if the patient weighs 100 pounds (approximately 45 kg), he/she would need 225 mg of medicine. Of course, as the MTE, it won't be up to you to make the calculation, just to type what the dictator said! And how do you do that?

Units of measurement are abbreviated in transcription—even if they are dictated in full (and they usually are). If you are transcribing two units of measurement, "mg" and "kg," and they are separated by the word *per*, you should also abbreviate the word *per*. Use a slash (/) to represent this small word. So, the example above would be transcribed:

5 mg/kg

One important rule to remember as relates to the term *per* is that if you are using the slash, you should always abbreviate the units of measurement. In pharmacology usage, you should be abbreviating units of measurement anyway, so this should be a pretty easy rule to internalize. However, you may see "per" in other contexts (such as speed). In those instances, the thing to keep in mind is consistency. It is perfectly acceptable to edit "miles per hour," or m/hr, but not miles/hour. Again, if you are using a slash, you will always abbreviate. If you are editing words in full, you should edit all the words in full.

Dictated	Correct	Incorrect
Fifteen milligrams per second	**15 mg/sec**	*15 mg per sec* *15 milligrams/second*
Sixty-two miles per hour	**62 m/hr**	*62 miles/hour* *62 m per hr*
One point five milligrams per kilogram	**1.5 mg/kg**	*1.5 milligrams/kilogram* *1.5 mg per kg*

Sometimes the word *per* can appear as part of an abbreviation, as in **parts per million** or **ppm**. This can either be dictated "ppm" or dictated in full, "parts per million." You should edit it according to the abbreviation, "ppm" and not p/m unless specifically indicated by your employer or account instructions.

One more thing about editing medication dosages before we move on: drugs are sometimes administered in amounts or percentages of less than 1. When editing such a dosage, you should always put a leading zero (0) and a decimal point. It helps to think of it this way—in a typed report, a decimal point by itself can be difficult to see. If a healthcare professional needed to refer to your report to determine a patient's dosage, and it was supposed to be, say ¼ of a cc or .25 cc, and the decimal point wasn't obvious...well...the results could be rather disastrous. Instead of getting ¼ of a cc, the patient would be given 25 cc, or 100 TIMES the proper dose! If it had been edited 0.25 cc, it would have been that much more obvious at first glance.

By the same token, where you should always add a leading zero and decimal to values less than one, you should never add a decimal point and zero for values greater than one. So, what does this look like?

Correct	Incorrect
0.25% lidocaine	*.25% lidocaine*
120 cc of fluid	*120.0 cc of fluid*

Multiple Choice.
Choose the correct way to edit each phrase.

1. Ten milligrams per kilogram

   ○ 10 mg/kg

   ○ 10 milligrams/kilogram

   ○ 10 mg per kg

2. Sixty-five miles per hour

   ○ 65 miles p hour

   ○ 65 m/hr

   ○ 65 miles/hour

3. One hundred parts per million

   ○ 100 parts/million

   ○ 100 parts p million

   ○ 100 ppm

4. Point-two-five percent Marcaine

   ○ .25% Marcaine

   ○ 0.25% Marcaine

   ○ 0.250% Marcaine

5. One thousand cubic centimeters of saline

   ○ 1000 cc saline

   ○ 1000.0 cc saline

   ○ 1000.00 cc saline

FREQUENCY

One element of a drug prescription—and a rather important element at that—is how often the patient is supposed to take a drug, also known as the frequency. Assume that you get the name of the drug right and the amount of the drug right, but not the drug frequency. Instead of once a day (q.d.), you have the patient taking it four times a day (q.i.d.)! Of course, if instructions were given in plain and simple English, this probably wouldn't be so difficult. After all, "four times a day" doesn't sound anything like "once a day," right?

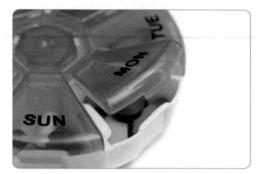

Well, this is medicalese, and we certainly wouldn't want to make it simple, so most drug instructions are given as Latin abbreviations. Furthermore, because they are abbreviations, they are dictated as a bunch of letters, sometimes a LOT of letters. Usually when a dictator gives you the amount of the drug "60 mg," he dictates it by saying the whole thing, "sixty milligrams." But when giving you the dosage instructions, it can be a big long string of random letters dictated one after the other. It becomes pretty important to understand what these letters mean and how they should be grouped. Let's take a look at some examples:

Dictated	Abbreviated From	Means
q.d.	quaque die	every day
q.i.d.	quater in die	four times a day
b.i.d.	bis in die	twice daily or two times a day
t.i.d.	ter in die	three times daily
h/hr	hora	hour

You do not need to know the Latin words; you will, however, need to know their English meanings.

Fill in the Blank.
Retype the abbreviation or the expansion in the blank provided.

1. d_____
2. day_____
3. b.i.d._____
4. twice daily or two times a day_____
5. h or hr_____
6. hour_____
7. t.i.d._____
8. three times daily_____
9. q.i.d._____
10. four times a day_____

Matching.
Match the appropriate terms below.

1. ____ b.i.d.   A. day
2. ____ t.i.d.   B. hour
3. ____ d   C. three times daily
4. ____ h   D. twice daily
5. ____ q.i.d.   E. four times a day

Multiple Choice.
Choose the best answer.

The patient was also followed by Dr. Stewart for depression and his lorazepam was increased to 2 mg t.i.d.

1. How often should the patient take lorazepam?

   ○ once a day

   ○ twice a day

   ○ three times a day

He will be discharged home on levofloxacin 350 mg p.o. b.i.d. for about 7 days.

2. How often should the patient take levofloxacin?

   ○ once a day

   ○ twice a day

   ○ three times a day

The patient was given 1000 cc initially, and it was allowed to run at 150 cc/h.

3. The patient's medication was given at a rate of 150 cc per:

   ○ second

   ○ minute

   ○ hour

He was diagnosed with hyperlipidemia. He is on Zocor 40 mg 1 p.o. d.

4. How often does the patient take Zocor for high cholesterol?

   ○ once a day

   ○ twice a day

   ○ three times a day

EVERY WHICH WAY

One letter that you will learn to love as you edit drug information is *q*. Although it isn't used much in everyday vernacular, in prescriptions it literally *means* "every," and it is used all the time. Abbreviated from the Latin word *quaque*, it is the primary means of designating frequency in prescriptions. So, whether the drug should be taken every day, every hour, every two hours, every four hours, or every other day, you are going to see the letter *q* appear.

Abbreviation	Meaning	
q.	every	
q.d.	every day	
q.h.	every hour *It's pretty uncommon for a drug to be taken every hour (although it does happen). But, you will see this all the time with the number of hours between doses, as follows. How these abbreviations are presented is a matter of style, to some extent. The general preference is to leave a space between the numeral and the unit of measurement. However, some accounts prefer no spaces. We may present the information a variety of acceptable ways throughout the program.*	
	q.2 h.	every two hours
	q.3 h.	every three hours
	q.4 h.	every four hours
	q.6 h.	every six hours
	q.8 h.	every eight hours
	q.12 h.	every twelve hours
q.h.s.	every bedtime or at bedtime	
q.i.d.*	four times a day	
q.o.d.	every other day	

*Technically speaking, this is not the same abbreviation as the rest of them. This stands for quater in die which means four times per day. From your perspective, though, a "q" is a "q!" Since you will not be typing the whole Latin words, you will just need to memorize what it stands for—just like the others.

Fill in the Blank.
Retype the abbreviation in the blank provided.

1. q.   _____

2. q.d.   _____

3. q.h.   _____

4. q.2 h.   _____

5. q.3 h.   _____

6. q.4 h.   _____

7. q.6 h.   _____

8. q.8 h.   _____

9. q.12 h.   _____

10. q.h.s.   _____

11. q.i.d.   _____

12. q.o.d.   _____

Matching.
Match the appropriate terms below.

1. ____ q.2 h.   A. every bedtime

2. ____ q.i.d.   B. every other day

3. ____ q.o.d.   C. every

4. ____ q.   D. every two hours

5. ____ q.d.   E. every day

6. ____ q.h.s.   F. four times a day

WHEN

You can now identify the amount of medication and the frequency with which it should be taken. Another component of the dosage instructions is when it should be taken. Believe it or not, this can make a huge difference in the efficacy of a drug. Here is an obvious example—you probably wouldn't want to take a sleeping medication first thing in the morning.

You may be aware from personal experience that there are a number of drugs which should not be taken on an empty stomach. Some antibiotics can cause stomach upset, even to the point of vomiting if taken without food. Other medications must be taken with water to make sure they travel all the way to your stomach and don't get stuck in your throat, instead. Even tiny pills can damage your esophagus if they dissolve before reaching your stomach.

So, when you take a drug can be an important component of the dosage instructions. Here are a few abbreviations you will need to know—the Latin meanings are just there for the sake of your curiosity.

Abbreviation	Meaning
a.c.	before meals or food (ante cibum)
a.m.	in the morning (ante meridiem)
h.s.	bedtime (hora somni)
p.m.	in the evening (post meridiem)
p.r.n.	as needed (pro re nata)

There are two ways that "p.r.n." will show up in the dosage instructions. First, is all by itself, just the abbreviation and you now know that means "as needed." Second, it can be used along with whatever it is needed for. So, an analgesic may be prescribed q.4-6 h. p.r.n. pain. That simply means that it should be taken every four to six hours as needed for pain. Whatever the indication or reason is for the medication could appear after p.r.n.—itching, cough, shortness of breath.

Fill in the Blank.
Retype the abbreviation or the expansion in the blank provided.

1. a.c._____
2. before meals or food_____
3. a.m._____
4. in the morning_____
5. h.s._____
6. bedtime_____
7. p.m._____
8. in the evening_____
9. p.r.n._____
10. as needed_____

Matching.
Match the appropriate terms below.

1. ____ p.m.   A. as needed
2. ____ h.s.   B. bedtime
3. ____ a.c.   C. in the morning
4. ____ p.r.n.   D. before food
5. ____ a.m.   E. in the evening

Proofreading.
Reformat the following longhand statements into abbreviated dosage instructions.

1. Acetaminophen elixir six-hundred and fifty milligrams every six hours as needed.

2. Amitriptyline ten milligrams at bedtime as needed.

3. Reglan ten milligrams before meals and at bedtime, four times a day.

4. Warfarin two milligrams every evening.

5. Glyburide five milligrams twice a day before meals.

6. Hydrocortisone ten milligrams, two tablets every morning and one tablet every evening.

WHERE AND WHERE ELSE

Although most drugs are taken orally, especially those prescribed by doctors for patients to take at home and on their own, there are other administration routes. Most of these you learned the English words for in an earlier unit. But it isn't enough that you know an otic suspension drop goes into the right ear, you also need to know that Latin phrase for the right ear. Or at least its Latin abbreviation. And even when the patient takes the drug by swallowing a pill or an elixir, the dosage instructions can't say it that simply. It, too, has its very own Latin phrase abbreviated to describe it.

Physicians can and do dictate the instructions using English words, i.e., saying "right eye" when they mean "right eye." However, they also frequently utilize these common Latin abbreviations when dictating dosage instructions. Go ahead and take note of the Latin terms, but don't worry too much about memorizing them. It may help you a little bit to notice that when it comes to the ear, the Latin word is aurio (think audio—it will help!) and when you're talking about the eye it's oculo. Thus, all ear abbreviations begin with *a* and all eye abbreviations begin with *o*.

As for the Latin abbreviation for taking a medication by mouth (p.o.), well, you may have already noticed its extremely frequent use. This is one that you will be editing so much you won't be able to imagine a time when you didn't know it.

Abbreviation	Meaning
a.d.	right ear *(aurio dextra)*
a.s.	left ear *(aurio sinister)*
a.u.	both ears *(aures utrae)*
o.d.	right eye *(oculus dexter)*
o.s.	left eye *(oculus sinister)*
o.u.	each eye *(oculo uterque)*
p.o.	by mouth *(per os)*

Fill in the Blank.
Retype the abbreviation in the blank provided.

1. a.d. _____

2. a.s. _____

3. a.u. _____

4. o.d. _____

5. o.s. _____

6. o.u. _____

7. p.o. _____

Matching.
Match the appropriate terms below.

1. ____ left eye   A. o.u.

2. ____ both ears   B. p.o.

3. ____ by mouth   C. a.s.

4. ____ right ear   D. o.s.

5. ____ each eye   E. a.u.

6. ____ right eye   F. o.d.

7. ____ left ear   G. a.d.

Fill in the Blank.
Enter the single letter that can represent each word.

1. Both   _____

2. Right   _____

3. Ear   _____

4. Left   _____

5. Eye   _____

6. Each   _____

TRUE TO FORM

There are a few other terms and abbreviations that will sometimes appear in dosage instructions that don't fit nicely into any of the above categories. Some of these should be familiar from earlier units in this module.

tab(s) from tablet(s): As you already know, the most common place a drug is administered is the mouth and the most common form it's in is a tablet. Physicians routinely dictate these as "tabs," and that's all that they mean.

EXAMPLES:

- Chlor-Trimeton-SR 8 mg 1 tab p.o. b.i.d. p.r.n
- He will be discharged on Bactrim single strength, 2 tabs p.o. b.i.d. times three days.

gtt from drops *(guttae)*: I would say that most dictators use the English word here, but you will see the Latin abbreviation. You had to figure that when they talked about putting medication o.u. or a.d. that those meds wouldn't be in pill form. Most dosages for the eyes and ears are measured in drops. This one really doesn't make a lot of sense, though, since the English drop is only one character longer, and drops is only two!

EXAMPLE:

- Restasis 1 gtt o.u. q.12 h.

MDI from metered dose inhaler: This is a delivery method for a common treatment of respiratory conditions. It is a device that delivers a specific premeasured dose of a medication in aerosol form to patients having difficulty breathing. Much like a dose of 10 mg of an oral pill would be called a "tab," doses on inhalers are called "puffs," and they will be dictated that way in the medical report.

EXAMPLES:

- Albuterol MDI p.r.n.
- Triamcinolone MDI 4 puffs b.i.d.

Fill in the Blank.
Retype the term or abbreviation in the blank provided.

1. tab(s)_____

2. tablet(s)_____

3. gtt_____

4. drops_____

5. MDI_____

6. metered dose inhaler_____

Fill in the Blank.
The following abbreviations and/or terms are used in the previous reports. Fill in the appropriate blank with either the abbreviation or its expansion.

1.MDI   _____

2.gtt   _____

3.tabs   _____

HAD ENOUGH?

There are just a few more terms that may appear in dosage instructions that you don't recognize at this point. Lots of the terms you have already learned in earlier units will come up as part of the instructions. Terms like *sublingual* (under the tongue), *suppositories* (a plug of medicine inserted somewhere other than the mouth), and *topically* (applied to the skin) are used to instruct how a medication is taken. Additionally, things like *extended-release* or *sustained-release* are used to describe the specific type of drug that is prescribed. And medication is sometimes given as a *bolus*—a single large dose of medication.

Sometimes drugs are **enteric-coated**. This coating allows the drug to pass through the stomach intact with the drug not being released until it is in the intestines. Can you think of why you may want this? There are three basic reasons:

1. To prevent destruction of the drug by stomach acid
2. To prevent stomach irritation
3. To delay onset of drug action

There is one more *q* abbreviation that you will see, but it doesn't have to do with "every." It turns out that in Latin, *q* is a pretty popular letter! The abbreviation **q.s.** is used occasionally in dosage instructions. It can mean one of two things:

- a sufficient quantity *(quantum sufficiat)*
- as much as is enough *(quantum satis)*

In pharmacology it can mean to add enough to fill the prescription—such as enough lactose to fill up the capsule. It can also be similar to the meaning of p.r.n., except it is related to how long the patient takes the drug instead of when the patient takes it.

One last thing that will appear in dosage instructions is the duration that the drug will be taken. There are many drugs that are not prescribed for a specific duration. For example, most diabetics that go on insulin can look forward to taking that drug for the rest of their lives. It's the same with cholesterol-lowering medication, thyroid pills, meds for high blood pressure, and so on.

On the other hand, lots and lots of drugs are used short term to treat a specific condition and then they are finished. Think antibiotics to knock out an infection, pain medication to treat an injury, or an antifungal cream to get rid of athlete's foot. In these instances, the dosage instructions should include either the finite time frame (duration or course) or the number of pills prescribed. There are a couple of different ways that physicians dictate these instructions.

Perhaps the most common is the word *times*, which literally means "a multiplicative word expressing the number of instances a thing occurs." This seems like a custom-tailored definition related to drug dosages because the dictator is, in elementary school math terms, using language to represent the mathematical symbol *x*.

The dictator says this:

"The patient has been prescribed Keflex 500 mg 1 p.o. t.i.d. **times seven days**."

There are a couple of different ways to edit this, and you will use the one that your employer or account instructions specifies. You can type it out longhand, as it appears above ("times seven days") or abbreviate it ("x 7 days" or "x7 days"). Some accounts prefer you leave a space between the *x* and numeral when dictated as "times," others prefer no space, and still others prefer you always insert the word "for" when the word *times* is used to represent duration. Of note, if a dictator uses the proper term and actually dictates "for" instead of "times" ("for seven days"), it is **not** appropriate to insert *x* or *times* instead.

Acceptable variation when dictated as "times seven days":

- Keflex 500 mg 1 p.o. t.i.d. times 7 days
- Keflex 500 mg 1 p.o. t.i.d. for 7 days
- Keflex 500 mg 1 p.o. t.i.d. x7 days
- Keflex 500 mg 1 p.o. t.i.d. x 7 days

Of note, some clients may also prefer numbers are spelled out, but the general trend is to use the numeral—although without specific instruction it would not necessarily be incorrect to edit as "seven."

Multiple Choice.
Choose the best answer.

1. The patient will be discharged on all previous medications, including Levaquin 500 mg p.o. q. day for four weeks. What are acceptable ways of editing the duration?

   ○ 4 4 weeks

   ○ for 4 weeks

   ○ x 4 weeks

   ○ times 4 weeks

   ○ all of the above

2. Clindamycin 300 mg p.o. q.i.d. times four weeks. How would you edit the duration?

   ○ times 4 w

   ○ X4W

   ○ times 4 weeks

3. The patient was prescribed _____-coated aspirin.

   ○ anteric

   ○ enteric

   ○ interic

   ○ intaric

4. Prevacid 30 mg p.o. q.d. on an empty stomach, x20. How long will the patient take the Prevacid?

   ○ 30 days

   ○ 25 days

   ○ 20 days

PUTTING IT ALL TOGETHER

Okay, now you have had all the fun of learning the dosage instructions one at a time. Let's see how much of it you assimilated. Read the following medication lists and answer the questions associated with them.

Multiple Choice.
Consult the following medication list for answers to the questions.

DISCHARGE MEDICATIONS:

1. Gabapentin 300 mg p.o. t.i.d.
2. Peri-Colace 1 p.o. b.i.d.
3. Albuterol power nebulizer q.6-8 h. p.r.n.
4. Theophylline 300 mg p.o. b.i.d.
5. Sertraline 50 mg p.o. q.d.
6. Multivitamin 1 p.o. q.d.
7. Combivent 2 puffs q.i.d.
8. Enteric-coated aspirin 325 mg p.o. q.d. (hold for two months due to bleeding).
9. Atenolol 50 mg p.o. q.d.
10. Ferrous sulfate 325 mg p.o. t.i.d.
11. Tylenol #3 1-2 p.o. q.6 h. p.r.n.
12. Alprazolam 0.5 mg p.o. t.i.d. p.r.n.

1. How often should the patient take Peri-Colace?

   ○ once a day

   ○ twice a day

   ○ three times a day

   ○ four times a day

2. How should the sertraline be taken?

   ○ as needed

   ○ for 50 days

   ○ by mouth

3. How often should the Combivent be taken?

   ○ once a day

   ○ twice a day

   ○ three times a day

   ○ four times a day

4. How often should the atenolol be taken?

   ○ once a day

   ○ twice a day

   ○ three times a day

   ○ four times a day

5. Which drug should be taken as needed three times a day?

- ○ atenolol
- ○ alprazolam
- ○ sertraline
- ○ albuterol

6. How much alprazolam should be taken?

- ○ 50 mg
- ○ 5 mg
- ○ 0.5 mg
- ○ 500 mg

7. How often should the gabapentin be taken?

- ○ once a day
- ○ twice a day
- ○ three times a day
- ○ four times a day

Fill in the Blank.
Consult the following medication list for answers to the questions.

Medical Record

DISCHARGE MEDICATIONS:

1. Lisinopril 20 mg p.o. q.d.
2. Isordil 40 mg p.o. t.i.d. with meals.
3. Temazepam 15 mg p.o. q.h.s. p.r.n.
4. Nitroglycerin sublingual tablets 0.4 mg p.r.n.
5. Colace 240 mg p.o. b.i.d. p.r.n.
6. Simvastatin 40 mg p.o. q.h.s.
7. Ranitidine 150 mg p.o. b.i.d.
8. Metoprolol 25 mg p.o. b.i.d.

---

1. Which drug is taken at bedtime, as needed?_____
2. Which drug is taken three times a day?_____
3. Which drug is taken in 25 mg doses twice a day?_____
4. Which drug is taken twice a day as needed?_____
5. Which drug is taken as needed, under the tongue?_____

Multiple Choice.
Consult the following medication list for answers to the questions.

DISCHARGE MEDICATIONS:

1. Amoxicillin 1 gm p.o. b.i.d. x 10 day course.
2. Diltiazem was discontinued.
3. Fosinopril was discontinued.
4. Lansoprazole 30 mg p.o. b.i.d. x 10 days, then 1 p.o. q.d.
5. Nitroglycerin sublingual p.r.n. q.5 minutes x3 for chest pain.
6. G-CSF 150 mcg subcu q.d. times 10 days.
7. Prednisone 100 mg p.o. q.d. times 2 days.
8. Tamoxifen 10 mg p.o. b.i.d.
9. Ciprofloxacin 250 mg p.o. b.i.d. for five weeks.
10. Metamucil 1 tbs p.o. q.a.m.
11. Ferrous sulfate 225 mg p.o. t.i.d. before meals.
12. Lopid 600 mg p.o. b.i.d.

1. What is the duration that the nitroglycerin should be taken?

   ○ as needed every 5 days

   ○ as needed every 3 days

   ○ as needed every 5 minutes

   ○ as needed every 5 minutes, 3 times

2. How many days should the patient take prednisone?

   ○ two

   ○ five

   ○ seven

   ○ ten

3. How often should the patient take ciprofloxacin?

   ○ once a day for five weeks

   ○ twice a day for five weeks

   ○ once a day for five days

   ○ twice a day for five days

4. What would another way be to represent the dosage instructions for ferrous sulfate?

   ○ 225 mg p.o. t.i.d. a.c.

   ○ 225 mg p.o. t.i.d. q.s.

   ○ 225 mg t.i.d. q.h.s.

5. What happens after ten days with the patient's lansoprazole?

   ○ it is discontinued

   ○ it drops to once a day

   ○ it goes up to three times a day

   ○ it stays at twice a day

6. How many mg of G-CSF is the patient supposed to take?

   ○ 0.15

   ○ 1.5

   ○ 150

   ○ 15.0

7. How much Metamucil should be taken and when?

   ○ 1 mg in the morning

   ○ 1 tablespoon in the morning

   ○ 1 tablespoon at bedtime

   ○ 1 mg at bedtime

8. What antibiotic will be taken by mouth, twice a day, for ten days?

   ○ Prednisone

   ○ Ciprofloxacin

   ○ Lansoprazole

   ○ Amoxicillin

UNIFORM USAGE

Technically speaking, everything that you have learned thus far about drug instructions is correct. No doubt about it, if you ask the "experts," this is the way to prescribe dosages, to "talk the talk." Now for the bad news. There is considerable variation in the dictation of drug dosage instructions, especially when it comes to frequency. Dictators may use the Latin abbreviations the way you just learned. They may also throw in an occasional English abbreviation or a mixture of Latin and English abbreviations. Just to totally confuse you, they may choose not to dictate any abbreviations at all!

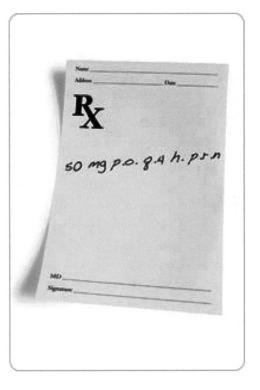

Let's take something simple. The patient is supposed to take a prescribed medication once a day, every day. You know this, you just learned it, right? It's q.d. But the dictator could say "daily," "q. daily," "once a day," or "every day." Sometimes, just to throw in a little redundancy, they'll say both, as in "q.d. every day."

What do you do?

First of all, it's never correct to be redundant. It's just redundant, repetitiously so. That one is easy. Eliminate the redundancy.

Really that is the only easy answer. What you do at this point really depends upon your employer or your account instructions. If you are instructed to edit only as dictated, then that is exactly what you do—mixed up language usage and everything. If the dictator says "q. daily," you edit to read "q. daily."

You may have account instructions to make things *consistent*, and they may even be so detailed as which way to make them specific: "use English" or "use the Latin abbreviation." Obviously these are easy instructions to follow. If your only guideline is to be consistent, then it will be up to you to pick the way that you like.

You may also be asked to make your dosage instructions consistent with abbreviated instructions versus spelled out ones. It is extremely unlikely that the majority of your dictation will consistently be done this way. Account instructions that require this kind of consistency would require you to make some significant changes to what is dictated. Here is a simple example:

Dictated: The patient is given 50 mg p.o. q.4 h. as needed.

If you as the MTE were going to make all of the instructions consistently abbreviated, then "as needed" should be changed to "p.r.n."

Made consistent: The patient is given 50 mg p.o. q.4 h. p.r.n.

There is no value judgment in this type of consistency. Remember, you are not writing a perfect document as an MTE. You are attempting to represent, as accurately as possible, the physician's dictation. There is no right or wrong way to making dosage instructions consistent. You just want to do whatever your employer or account instructions tell you to. In this career, you won't win any brownie points by telling your client or employer what the right way is and ignoring their preferences or instructions. And the reality is that you will edit dosage instructions differently in different situations.

Finally, there may be a factor of whether what was dictated qualifies as a "dangerous abbreviation," which can happen with or without mixing up the English and Latin. We will deal with that a little later, but for now the important rules are:

- Don't be redundant.
- Follow your account instructions.
- Be consistent.

MULTIPLE CHOICE.
Read the following excerpt and answer the questions.

The terazosin will be changed to 4 mg p.o. at h.s. daily, and his blood pressures will be checked.

1. How and how frequently will the patient be taking his terazosin?

   ○ by mouth, once a day, at bedtime

   ○ by mouth, once a day, in the morning

   ○ by mouth, every hour, at bedtime

   ○ intravenously, every hour, every day

2. Assume your account instructions are "exactly as dictated." What changes would you make to the dosage instructions?

   ○ 4 mg p.o. q. bedtime

   ○ 4 mg p.o. q.h.s.

   ○ 4 mg by mouth h.s. daily

   ○ no changes

3. Assume your account instructions are to make it consistent, using the Latin abbreviations. How can you change the dosage instructions using the fewest keystrokes?

   ○ 4 mg p.o. q. bedtime

   ○ 4 mg p.o. q.h.s.

   ○ 4 mg by mouth h.s. daily

   ○ 4 mg p.o. at h.s. daily

4. The patient has hyperlipidemia. He is on Zocor 40 mg 1 p.o. q. day. How could you change the dictation to make it consistent?

   ○ Zocor 40 mg 1 p.o. q.d.

   ○ Zocor 40 mg 1 p.o. daily

   ○ Both are correct

5. Choose the correct dosage instructions.

   ○ Salsalate 750 mg t.i.d. a.c. with meals.

   ○ Salsalate 750 mg t.i.d. with meals.

   ○ Salsalate 750 mg t.i.d. a.c.

PROOFREADING.
Make the following dosage instructions consistent using Latin abbreviations.

1. Refill enteric-coated aspirin 325 mg p.o. q.day.

2. Pseudoephedrine 30 mg p.o. q. six hours p.r.n.

3. Timolol solution b.i.d. in the right eye, 1 drop.

4. Atenolol 50 mg p.o. q.d. daily.

DANGEROUS ABBREVIATIONS

The Institute for Safe Medication Practices (ISMP) is a nonprofit organization based in Pennsylvania. They exist to help prevent medication error and ensure the safe use of medications. Their website states their mission to be:

OUR MISSION

To advance patient safety worldwide by empowering the healthcare community, including consumers, to prevent medication errors.

We accomplish this through our interdisciplinary efforts to:

- Collect and analyze reports of medication-related hazardous conditions, near-misses, errors, and other adverse drug events.
- Disseminate timely medication safety information, risk-reduction tools, and error-prevention strategies.
- Educate the healthcare community and consumers about safe medication practices.
- Collaborate with other patient safety organizations, educational institutions, governmental agencies and other healthcare stakeholders.
- Advocate the adoption of safe medication standards by accrediting bodies, manufacturers, policy makers, regulatory agencies, and standards-setting organizations.
- Conduct research to provide evidence-based safe medication practices.

So, how do they accomplish this, and what does it have to do with medical transcription editing?

It has been the determination of the ISMP that there are some abbreviations which have been/are consistently used in medical reporting which are easily or frequently misinterpreted and could therefore potentially result in harmful medication errors. Furthermore, they maintain that these abbreviations should never be used when communicating medical information in any way (particularly in typed records). Many of these "dangerous abbreviations" are the very abbreviations that you just spent so much time learning!

Dangerous abbreviations include such things as a.d., a.s., and a.u., which they maintain can easily be mistaken for each other. Other "dangerous abbreviations" include h.s., q.o.d., and IU. For the most part, their recommendation to correct a dangerous abbreviation is to spell it out in English: right eye, left eye, each eye, bedtime, every other day, and (in the case of international units) units.

It seems reasonable, don't you think? The problem is that you will receive explicit account instructions that contradict the recommendations of the ISMP. In these instances, just as everywhere else in your career as an MTE, you should do what your employer tells you to do. Sometimes, however, those account instructions will include correcting for dangerous abbreviations.

Following is a link to their list of dangerous abbreviations. You can also do a search by their organization name (ISMP) to find them on the Internet. In any case, if you are explicitly instructed to correct dangerous abbreviations, verify what qualifies and make the appropriate changes.

Career Step is not affiliated with the Institute for Safe Medication Practices. The Institute for Safe Medication Practices is just one of many good sources available and is used here for illustrative purposes.

ANSWER KEY

TWO TYPES OF DRUGS

I. MULTIPLE CHOICE.

Over-the-counter
behind-the-counter
behind-the-counter

2. over-the-counter
4. prescription

DRUG NAMES

II. MULTIPLE CHOICE.

three
rarely
never

2. always
4. trade or brand

DRUG EFFECT

II. MULTIPLE CHOICE.

local
local
systemic

2. systemic
4. local

Administration

TOPICAL, ENTERAL, AND PARENTERAL

II. MATCHING.

A. topical

B. enteral

B. enteral

D. transdermal

2. B. enteral

4. C. parenteral

6. C. parenteral OR D. transdermal

8. B. enteral

TOPICAL – EARS AND EYES

I. MATCHING.

B. ophthalmic

C. both

B. ophthalmic

A. otic

B. ophthalmic

2. B. ophthalmic

4. B. ophthalmic

6. C. both

8. B. ophthalmic

10. C. both

TOPICAL – DENTAL AND INHALATION

I. TRUE/FALSE.

false

true

2. true

4. true

II. SPELLING.

lidocaine

carbamide peroxide

Xylocaine

2. Citanest

4. inhalation

TOPICAL – SKIN AND NOSE

I. MATCHING.

A. skin

A. skin

B. nose

2. B. nose

4. A. skin

TOPICAL – VAGINAL

I. TRUE/FALSE.

true

true

2. false

4. false

REVIEW: TOPICAL

I. MATCHING.

C. inserted into the vagina

B. inside the eye

E. tightens blood vessels

2. D. pertaining to the ear

4. A. breathed in

II. SPELLING.

corticosteroids

Neosporin

benzocaine

TobraDex

Mydriacyl

2. Monistat

4. Afrin

6. albuterol

8. potassium chloride

ENTERAL METHODS

II. MULTIPLE CHOICE.
enteral
Dulcolax
glycerine OR glycerin

2. oral
4. bisacodyl

ENTERAL FORMS

PARENTERAL – IN THE MOUTH

I. MATCHING.
E. under the tongue
D. a narcotic
A. in the cheek

2. B. can be penetrated
4. C. relaxes blood vessels

II. MULTIPLE CHOICE.
buccal
Subutex
sublingual

2. permeable
4. buprenorphine SL
6. isosorbide dinitrate SL

PARENTERAL – BREATHING IT IN

I. TRUE/FALSE.
true

2. true

PARENTERAL – INTRAVENOUS INJECTIONS

I. MATCHING.
B. intravenous
A. a small device for injecting fluids

2. C. needle diameter

II. MULTIPLE CHOICE.
22 gauge

PARENTERAL – STILL INJECTING IT

I. MATCHING.
C. single, large dose
B. total parenteral nutrition

2. A. peripherally inserted central catheter

II. MULTIPLE CHOICE.
intravenous drip
total parenteral nutrition
PICC

2. bolus
4. central IV line

PARENTERAL – OTHER WAYS

I. MULTIPLE CHOICE.
subcutaneous
intravenous
intramuscular

2. intramuscular
4. subcutaneous

REVIEW: ENTERAL AND PARENTERAL

I. TRUE/FALSE.
true
false

2. true
4. false

II. MATCHING.
C. nasogastric
E. intravenous
G. gastrostomy
B. under the skin

2. A. inhalational
4. H. single, large dose
6. D. in the muscle
8. F. spinal injection

Drug Categories

ANTIARRHYTHMICS

I. TRUE/FALSE.
true

false

false

2. true

4. true

II. MULTIPLE CHOICE.
metoprolol

procainamide

Procan SR

Lopressor

2. amiodarone

4. disopyramide

6. mexiletine

8. Pronestyl

ANTICOAGULANTS

II. MULTIPLE CHOICE.
anticoagulant

heparin

Lovenox

2. warfarin

4. thrombolytic

I. SPELLING.
heparin

thrombolytics

Lovenox

2. anticoagulants

4. Coumadin

ANTIHYPERLIPIDEMICS

I. MATCHING.
E. Questran

F. TriCor

G. Zocor

A. Colestid

2. D. Mevacor

4. B. Lipitor

6. C. Lopid

II. MULTIPLE CHOICE.
Mevacor

atorvastatin

Lipitor

colestipol

gemfibrozil

2. fenofibrate

4. Lopid

6. cholestyramine

8. simvastatin

10. niacin

ANTIHYPERTENSIVES

I. TRUE/FALSE.
false

true

false

2. false

4. true

II. MATCHING.
C. Catapres

B. Capoten

E. Vasotec

2. D. Monopril

4. A. Aldoril

6. F. Zestril

VASODILATORS

I. MULTIPLE CHOICE.

phentolamine

vasodilators

Nitro-Bid

hydralazine

nitroglycerin

2. minoxidil

4. prazosin

6. isosorbide

8. Imdur

10. Apresoline

BETA BLOCKERS

I. MULTIPLE CHOICE.

all kinds of tremors

Timolol

slower heart rate

2. carvedilol

4. adrenaline

II. SPELLING.

Inderal

propranolol

carvedilol

2. metoprolol

4. Betimol

CALCIUM CHANNEL BLOCKERS

I. TRUE/FALSE.

Calan

Norvasc

Procardia

verapamil

2. nifedipine

4. diltiazem

6. amlodipine

8. Cardizem

REVIEW: CARDIOVASCULAR DRUGS

I. MULTIPLE CHOICE.

adrenaline

antihypertensive

antiarrhythmics

2. hypotension

4. lipid-lowering agents

II. SPELLING.

metoprolol

Coumadin

simvastatin

warfarin

Vasotec

isosorbide

nitroglycerin

atenolol

2. Lopressor

4. Lipitor

6. Mevacor

8. Zestril

10. enalapril

12. diltiazem

14. propranolol

ANTACIDS – LESSON 1

I. MULTIPLE CHOICE.

all of the above

calcium

Tums

ALternaGEL

Rolaids

2. laxative

4. magnesium

6. Maalox

8. magnesium

ANTACIDS – LESSON 2

I. MULTIPLE CHOICE.

nizatidine
famotidine
cimetidine
Prilosec
Pepcid AC

2. sucralfate
4. lansoprazole
6. Tagamet
8. ranitidine
10. Prevacid

ANTIEMETICS

I. TRUE/FALSE.

false
true
true
true
false

2. true
4. false
6. false
8. false
10. true

II. MULTIPLE CHOICE.

scopolamine
Tigan
meclizine

2. antiemetics
4. Pepto-Bismol

REVIEW: DIGESTIVE DRUGS

I. MULTIPLE CHOICE.

neutralizing
calcium carbonate
sucralfate
vomit
meclizine

2. histamines
4. cimetidine
6. brain
8. antiemetics
10. Tigan

II. TRUE/FALSE.

true
false
true
true
false

2. false
4. true
6. true
8. true
10. false

DIURETICS

I. MULTIPLE CHOICE.

increase
kidneys
decreases

2. take water out of
4. furosemide

II. SPELLING.

hydrochlorothiazide
spironolactone
furosemide

2. Lasix
4. Aldactone

DIABETES

I. MATCHING.
C. juvenile diabetes
E. occurs during pregnancy

F. adult-onset diabetes mellitus

2. A. stimulates the liver to release glucose
4. B. secreted by the pancreas to regulate glucose
6. D. disease where the body cannot make or use insulin

II. FILL IN THE BLANK.
insulin-dependent diabetes mellitus
adult OR adult-
juvenile

gestational

2. insulin
4. glucagon
6. mellitus
8. non insulin-dependent diabetes mellitus OR noninsulin-dependent diabetes mellitus

DIABETIC MEDICATIONS

INSULIN

I. MULTIPLE CHOICE.
type 1 and type 2 diabetes
Rapid-acting
subcutaneously

2. lowers
4. 12-18

II. MATCHING.
C. Novolog
B. Humalog
A. Humulin

2. A. Humulin
4. A. Humulin

THYROID HORMONES

I. TRUE/FALSE.
false
true
false

2. true
4. false

II. SPELLING.
levothyroxine
Levoxyl
Synthroid

2. propylthiouracil
4. Cytomel

SEX HORMONES

I. MULTIPLE CHOICE.
Depo-Provera
Ortho-Novum
Ortho Tri-Cyclen
progesterone

2. estrogen
4. testosterone
6. Lybrel

PREGNANCY AND HORMONES

I. MULTIPLE CHOICE.
more
Oxytocin
Estrogen
Pitocin
labor

2. Human chorionic gonadotropin
4. induces
6. Pitocin
8. Cytotec

INFERTILITY AND HORMONES

I. MULTIPLE CHOICE.

clomiphene
Clomid
sex hormones

2. Estradiol
4. decrease

REVIEW: ENDOCRINE DRUGS

I. MATCHING.

F. Humulin
A. Glucophage
G. Pregnyl
D. Aldactone
J. Clomid

2. I. Ortho Tri-Cyclen
4. E. Lasix
6. C. Synthroid
8. H. Pitocin
10. B. Micronase

II. TRUE/FALSE.

true
false
false

2. true
4. true

PENICILLINS

CEPHALOSPORINS

I. SPELLING.

cefuroxime
ceftriaxone
Rocephin

2. Keflex
4. ceftazidime

MACROLIDES AND TETRACYCLINE

I. MULTIPLE CHOICE.

Macrolides
proteins
decreased

2. doxycycline
4. Tetracycline

II. MATCHING.

A. macrolides
B. tetracyclines
B. tetracyclines

2. B. tetracyclines
4. A. macrolides
6. A. macrolides

QUINOLONES AND OTHER ANTIBIOTICS

I. MULTIPLE CHOICE.

Cipro
metronidazole
vancomycin
Neosporin

2. bacitracin
4. Flagyl
6. polymyxin B
8. Garamycin

ANTIVIRALS AND ANTIFUNGALS

I. TRUE/FALSE.

false
true
false
true
true

2. false
4. false
6. true
8. false
10. false

CYTOTOXICS

I. MULTIPLE CHOICE.

Adriamycin
doxorubicin
ifosfamide
Oncovin

2. Trexall
4. methotrexate
6. vincristine

REVIEW: IMMUNE DRUGS

I. MULTIPLE CHOICE.

antibiotics
tetracycline
vancomycin
chemotherapy

2. cephalosporin
4. ciprofloxacin
6. antiretroviral
8. immunosuppressives

II. TRUE/FALSE.

false
true
true

2. true
4. true

NON-NARCOTIC ANALGESICS

I. TRUE/FALSE.

false
false
true

2. true
4. false

II. SPELLING.

Naprosyn
ibuprofen
aspirin

2. Bayer
4. nonsteroidal

NSAIDS

I. MATCHING.

E. Voltaren
C. Relafen
D. Tolectin

2. B. Indocin
4. A. Feldene

II. SPELLING.

naproxen
Feldene
nabumetone

2. inflammatory
4. Nuprin

NARCOTIC ANALGESICS

II. MULTIPLE CHOICE.

Percocet
OxyContin
Vicodin
Darvon
Demerol

2. Tylox
4. Percodan
6. Lorcet
8. Ultram
10. MS-Contin

ANESTHESIA

I. MULTIPLE CHOICE.

procaine
anesthesia
lidocaine
Xylocaine
Diprivan

2. nitrous oxide
4. methohexital
6. Orajel
8. midazolam
10. Versed

CORTICOSTEROIDS

I. MULTIPLE CHOICE.

arthritis

-olone

cortisol

2. for a limited time

4. hydrocortisone

II. MATCHING.

D. Luxiq

B. Decadron

C. Kenalog

2. A. Cortone Acetate

4. E. Medrol

REVIEW: PAIN MANAGEMENT DRUGS

I. FILL IN THE BLANK.

opium

inflammation

local

corticosteroids

2. nonsteroidal

4. narcotics

6. amnesic

8. prednisone

II. MATCHING.

A. Aleve

I. Cortone Acetate

B. Tolectin

E. Ultram

D. Xylocaine

2. G. Tylenol

4. F. Excedrin

6. H. Relafen

8. C. MS-Contin

10. J. Versed

ANTIANXIETY

I. MULTIPLE CHOICE.

benzodiazepines

Xanax

BuSpar

Klonopin

Halcion

2. buspirone

4. Valium

6. buspirone

8. Flexeril

10. antianxiety medications

ANTIDEPRESSANTS

I. MULTIPLE CHOICE.

all of the above

increasing

selective serotonin reuptake inhibitors

2. short-term 'blues'

4. potentially lethal

II. MATCHING.

B. SSRI

A. tricyclic

B. SSRI

2. D. tetracyclic and others

4. B. SSRI

ANTIPSYCHOTICS

I. SPELLING.

haloperidol

chlorpromazine

lithium

Thorazine

2. risperidone

4. olanzapine

6. clozapine

8. Haldol

REVIEW: PSYCHOLOGICAL DRUGS

I. MULTIPLE CHOICE.
Benzodiazepines
neuroleptics
antianxiety

2. serotonin
4. chemicals

II. TRUE/FALSE.
true
false
true

2. true
4. true

ANTIHISTAMINES

I. MULTIPLE CHOICE.
schizophrenia
play a role in digestion
anxiolytic
acetaminophen or other additional drugs
brompheniramine

2. antiemetics
4. diphenhydramine
6. Allegra
8. cetirizine
10. Claritin

BRONCHODILATORS

I. MULTIPLE CHOICE.
bronchodilator
Slo-bid
Serevent
Combivent
ipratropium

2. Proventil
4. beta-agonist
6. albuterol
8. theophylline

COUGH SUPPRESSANTS AND EXPECTORANTS

I. TRUE/FALSE.
Chloraseptic
guaifenesin
menthol

2. antitussives
4. dextromethorphan
6. expectorant

DECONGESTANTS

I. MULTIPLE CHOICE.
stuffy nose
Pseudoephedrine
nasally

2. slowly
4. constricting blood vessels

II. SPELLING.
pseudoephedrine
decongestant
phenylephrine

2. Dristan
4. Sudafed

REVIEW: RESPIRATORY DRUGS

I. FILL IN THE BLANK.
antiemetics
Beta-agonists OR Short-acting beta agonists
Decongestants

2. Benadryl
4. Codeine

II. MULTIPLE CHOICE.
neurotransmitter
Theophylline
pseudoephedrine

2. asthma
4. expectorant

Using References

EPOCRATES.COM

I. FILL IN THE BLANK.
atorvastatin OR atorvastatin calcium
heart attack
seizures

2. cholesterol
4. pregabalin
6. nerve

DRUGS.COM

I. MULTIPLE CHOICE.
insomnia
Antivert
XL

2. anticholinergic
4. diuretic

EXPRESS SCRIPTS

I. MULTIPLE CHOICE.
salmeterol aerosol inhalation
Zestril

2. type 2 diabetes
4. brand name

FDA.GOV

I. MULTIPLE CHOICE.
500 mg
tablet
metoprolol

2. metformin hydrochloride
4. Tirosint

WEBMD.COM

I. FILL IN THE BLANK.
anxiety
Prilosec OR Prilosec OTC

2. Procardia

II. MULTIPLE CHOICE.
furosemide

GENERAL LOOK-UPS

IT ALL LOOKS A LITTLE FUZZY

I. MULTIPLE CHOICE.
Norvasc

II. FILL IN THE BLANK.
Prevacid
felodipine

2. lansoprazole
4. Tenormin

KNOW THE DOSE

I. FILL IN THE BLANK.
Zantac

2. ranitidine

II. MULTIPLE CHOICE.
25 mg
50 mg

2. 0.1 mg

THE RIGHT CONDITION

SOUNDS LIKE, BUT NOT QUITE

WOULD YOU LIKE SOME HERBS WITH THAT?

I. MULTIPLE CHOICE.

Mythical Bush

Hamamelis viginiana

2. hemorrhoids

GOING STRAIGHT TO THE HORSE\'S MOUTH

I. MULTIPLE CHOICE.

insulin

lower cholesterol

2. KwikPen

4. atorvastatin calcium

SAY WHAT?!

I. MULTIPLE CHOICE.

Flag it

Flag it

It's fine

2. It's fine

4. Flag it

Formatting

UNITS OF MEASUREMENT

I. FILL IN THE BLANK.

gram	2. g
kilogram	4. kg
milligram	6. mg
microgram	8. mcg
International Unit	10. IU

II. MATCHING.

C. microgram	2. D. gram
A. International Unit	4. E. milligram
B. kilogram	

IV. MULTIPLE CHOICE.

base 10	2. 100 mg
only in units of measurement	4. 12,000
milligrams	

THE METRIC SYSTEM

II. FILL IN THE BLANK.

milliequivalents	2. cubic centimeter
l	4. mL
kcal	6. liter
kilocalorie	8. milliliter
mEq	10. cc

MEASURING UP IN THE USA

II. FILL IN THE BLANK.

pound	2. fl oz
teaspoon	4. lb
ounce	6. oz
fluid ounce	8. tsp

PER-PER-PERFECT ZERO

I. MULTIPLE CHOICE.

10 mg/kg	2. 65 m/hr
100 ppm	4. 0.25% Marcaine
1000 cc saline	

FREQUENCY

II. MATCHING.

D. twice daily	2. C. three times daily
A. day	4. B. hour
E. four times a day	

III. MULTIPLE CHOICE.

three times a day	2. twice a day
hour	4. once a day

EVERY WHICH WAY

II. MATCHING.

D. every two hours

B. every other day

E. every day

2. F. four times a day

4. C. every

6. A. every bedtime

WHEN

II. MATCHING.

E. in the evening

D. before food

C. in the morning

2. B. bedtime

4. A. as needed

III. PROOFREADING.

1. Acetaminophen elixir ~~six hundred and fifty milligrams every six hours as needed~~ **650 mg q.6 h. p.r.n.**
2. Amitriptyline ~~ten milligrams at bedtime as needed~~ **10 mg h.s. p.r.n.**
3. Reglan ~~ten milligrams before meals~~ **10 mg a.c.** and ~~at bedtime, four times a day~~ **h.s. q.i.d.**
4. Warfarin ~~two milligrams every evening~~ **2 mg q.p.m.**
5. Glyburide ~~five milligrams twice a day before meals~~ **5 mg b.i.d. a.c.**
6. Hydrocortisone ~~ten milligrams~~ **10 mg,** ~~two tablets every morning and one tablet every evening~~ **2 tabs q.a.m., 1 tab q.p.m.**

WHERE AND WHERE ELSE

II. MATCHING.

D. o.s.

B. p.o.

A. o.u.

C. a.s.

2. E. a.u.

4. G. a.d.

6. F. o.d.

III. FILL IN THE BLANK.

U

A

O

2. D

4. S

6. U

TRUE TO FORM

II. FILL IN THE BLANK.

metered dose inhaler

tablets

2. drops

HAD ENOUGH?

I. MULTIPLE CHOICE.

for 4 weeks

enteric

2. times 4 weeks

4. 20 days

PUTTING IT ALL TOGETHER

I. MULTIPLE CHOICE.

twice a day
four times a day
Alprazolam
three times a day

2. by mouth
4. once a day
6. 0.5 mg

II. FILL IN THE BLANK.

temazepam
Metoprolol
Nitroglycerin

2. Isordil
4. Colace

III. MULTIPLE CHOICE.

as needed every 5 minutes, 3 times
twice a day for five weeks
it drops to once a day
1 tablespoon in the morning

2. two
4. 225 mg p.o. t.i.d. a.c.
6. 0.15 OR .15
8. Amoxicillin

UNIFORM USAGE

I. MULTIPLE CHOICE.

by mouth, once a day, at bedtime
4 mg p.o. q.h.s.
Salsalate 750 mg t.i.d. with meals. OR Salsalate 750
mg t.i.d. a.c.

2. no changes
4. Both are correct

II. PROOFREADING.

1. Refill enteric-coated aspirin 325 mg p.o. ~~q.day~~ **q.d.**

2. Pseudoephedrine 30 mg p.o. ~~q~~ **q.6 h.** ~~six hours~~ p.r.n.

3. Timolol solution b.i.d. ~~in the right eye,~~ **o.d.** 1 ~~drop~~ **gtt.**

4. Atenolol 50 mg p.o. q.d ~~.daily~~.